# Testimonials for the
## *The Keys to Your Health*

"People are becoming more and more aware of the different choices they can make about their health and Janice Alexander is eager to spread the word far and wide and makes it easy for people to understand how they can take more responsibility and empower themselves in a way that gives them confidence to take their health in their hands."

—Sharon Smith
author of *Eat Your Way to Health and Wellbeing*

"A timely book. Janice has managed to engage those of us who for years have managed to avoid taking stock of what we eat and the impact on our health. Her book is a great source of the good, the bad and ugly in food. It's a great reference on how to transition from a dead diet to one of life and vitality."

—Vivienne Springer-Williams
Parenting Coach

"Janice Alexander is the real deal, in this book she has translated her own life experiences and comprehensive studies of the field of health and nutrition into sensible and practical guidelines for creating a vibrant and healthful life. A must read for everyone who is serious about vital living."

—Michael Don Smith
Business strategy master coach.

8 Secrets to
Long and Vital Living

# THE KEYS
## to
# YOUR HEALTH

**JANICE ALEXANDER** Bsc (Hons)
Health Practice (Osteopathy) degree
Health Restore Advanced Programme
Nutrition Certificate Stage 3

First Edition Published by Janice Alexander

www.TheKeysToYourHealth.com

Copyright ©2018 Janice Alexander

ISBN-13: 978-1983680762

All rights reserved. Neither this book, nor any parts within it may be sold or reproduced in any form without permission.

No part of this book may be reproduced in any form or by any electronic or mechanical means including information storage and retrieval systems, without permission in writing from the author. The only exception is by a reviewer, who may quote short excerpts in a review.

# Dedication

This book is dedicated to you, the reader.

The reason I decided to write this book was because I know that people want to be healthy and don't know how. They just want to have the knowledge to be able to prevent ill health or even turn around any health challenges they might have and to live a long life that is vital and energetic and really healthy so that living to one hundred and beyond is a desirable prospect rather than something to fear. Healthy means that you have all your faculties, you are firing on all cylinders; your eyesight is clear, your ears can hear, your brain is as sharp as a razor, you have a spring in your step, have no pain and have plenty of energy. Janice Alexander with love.

# Contents

About the Author ........................................................... xiii
Foreword ........................................................................ xiv
Acknowledgments .......................................................... xv
Note to the reader ......................................................... xvi

1. Define What Health Is ............................................... 1
    1.1   Healthy at 90 ................................................... 1
    1.2   Old age doesn't mean unhealthy ...................... 2
    1.3   Epigenetics ...................................................... 2
    1.4   The way we live makes a difference ................. 3
    1.5   Inflammatory foods cause problems ................ 4
    1.6   Drugs cause epigenetic diseases ...................... 5
    1.7   The organs work in sync .................................. 7
    1.8   Your body is always talking to you .................. 7

2. Water .......................................................................... 9
    2.1   Water is life ..................................................... 9
    2.2   Dehydration dangers ..................................... 10
    2.3   What water should we drink? ........................ 11

|      |      |                                                              |
|------|------|--------------------------------------------------------------|
|      | 2.4  | Machines that treat water ....................................12 |
|      | 2.5  | No to tap water .......................................13     |
|      | 2.6  | We don't want plastic water ....................14           |
|      | 2.7  | We definitely need a filter ......................14         |
| 3.   | The Micro Biome ..............................................17 |                                                              |
|      | 3.1  | Health starts with the gut ......................17          |
|      | 3.2  | Micro biome: What is it? ........................18          |
|      | 3.3  | Where do we get our microbes from? ...19                     |
|      | 3.4  | Does it all boil down to your genes? ........20              |
|      | 3.5  | Three billion bacteria are shared from the mouth to the gut every day .........21 |
|      | 3.6  | Stress affects your micro biome ...............22            |
|      | 3.7  | The gut connection to Alzheimer's .........23                |
|      | 3.8  | Brains are made of saturated fat .............24             |
|      | 3.9  | The role of the gut in colitis ....................25        |
|      | 3.10 | Faecal transplants work ..........................25         |
|      | 3.11 | Xenoestrogen's can cause breast cancer ....26                |
|      | 3.12 | You are in control of your micro biome ...27                 |
| 4.   | Are We Designed To Eat meat? ...................................29 |                                                              |
|      | 4.1  | What are we designed to eat? ...............29               |
|      | 4.2  | Gathering the evidence ..........................30          |
|      | 4.3  | Who told you they were canines? ...........34                |
| 5.   | Sleep ..........................................................39 |                                                              |
|      | 5.1  | What is the point of sleep? ....................39           |
|      | 5.2  | Insomnia can cause diabetes ..................40             |

| | 5.3 | How much sleep is enough sleep? | 41 |
|---|---|---|---|
| | 5.4 | How lack of sleep causes disease | 42 |
| | 5.5 | How we set our natural body clock | 42 |
| | 5.6 | How to get beauty sleep | 43 |
| | 5.7 | Light is important for well being | 43 |
| | 5.8 | Electromagnetic radiation ionizes our cells | 44 |
| | 5.9 | Child night lights linked to depression | 45 |
| | 5.10 | Deep sleep | 46 |
| | 5.11 | We need melatonin to sleep | 47 |
| | 5.12 | When is the best time to sleep? | 48 |
| | 5.13 | What's the best temperature for sleep? | 48 |
| 6. | Looking After The Terrain | | 49 |
| | 6.1 | Terrain is built on pH balance | 49 |
| | 6.2 | Low pH and calcium | 50 |
| | 6.3 | Dangers of artificial sugars | 51 |
| | 6.4 | Dangers of using a microwave | 52 |
| | 6.5 | The germ theory | 53 |
| | 6.6 | Starting from the beginning | 53 |
| | 6.7 | Feeding baby the best | 54 |
| | 6.8 | Normal birth colonization | 55 |
| | 6.9 | Milk is species specific | 56 |
| | 6.10 | Listen to your biological clock | 57 |
| | 6.11 | Avoiding chemicals | 59 |
| | 6.12 | Non-food, food | 59 |
| | 6.13 | Unclog the organs | 60 |
| | 6.14 | Alternative to antibiotics | 60 |
| | 6.15 | Why we don't want Wi-Fi | 61 |

|      |      |                                              |
|------|------|----------------------------------------------|
|      | 6.16 | Toxic air in your home ......................... 62 |
|      | 6.17 | If you can't eat it, forget it ................. 62 |
|      | 6.18 | Clean up your bedroom ........................ 63 |
|      | 6.19 | Our clothes can kill us ........................ 64 |
| 7.   | Vitamin D ............................................................ 67 |     |
|      | 7.1  | Importance of Vitamin D .................... 67 |
|      | 7.2  | Vitamin D is a hormone ...................... 67 |
|      | 7.3  | How do we get hormone D? ............... 69 |
| 8.   | Exercise .............................................................. 71 |     |
|      | 8.1  | Exercise, can you be healthy without it? ........ 71 |
|      | 8.2  | Exercise benefits the muscles ............. 72 |
|      | 8.3  | Exercise is good for the joints ............ 73 |
|      | 8.4  | Exercise is good for the nerves .......... 73 |
|      | 8.5  | Sitting is the new smoking ................. 74 |
|      | 8.6  | Is sleeping bad too? ............................. 77 |
|      | 8.7  | Exercise and the micro biome ............ 78 |
|      | 8.8  | Exercise slows ageing .......................... 78 |
|      | 8.9  | Exercise helps dementia ..................... 79 |
|      | 8.10 | How to reduce your sitting time ........ 80 |
|      | 8.11 | Breathing for vitality ........................... 81 |
| 9.   | Fasting ............................................................... 83 |     |
|      | 9.1  | What is fasting? ................................... 83 |
|      | 9.2  | Why would anyone want to get into ketosis? ... 85 |
|      | 9.3  | Carbohydrates and gaining weight ..... 87 |
|      | 9.4  | Benefits of calorie restriction ............. 87 |

| | | |
|---|---|---|
| 9.5 | The many different ways of fasting | 88 |
| 9.6 | Benefits of a detox | 89 |

## 10. Putting it all together ... 93

| | | |
|---|---|---|
| 10.1 | Giving the body what it needs | 93 |
| 10.2 | The importance of hydration | 94 |
| 10.3 | Strengthen the terrain | 95 |
| 10.4 | Watch those toxic dental procedures | 95 |
| 10.5 | Hormone D protects your health | 96 |
| 10.6 | Getting a great night sleep | 96 |
| 10.7 | Get the right equipment | 97 |
| 10.8 | Bye bye to processed food | 98 |
| 10.9 | Processed food and low fertility | 99 |
| 10.10 | No irradiation thank you | 99 |
| 10.11 | Toxic air in your house | 100 |
| 10.12 | Swop out the chemicals | 101 |
| 10.13 | Swop out your Wi-Fi | 102 |
| 10.14 | Toxic clothes | 102 |
| 10.15 | Exercise | 103 |
| 10.16 | Detoxify or die | 103 |
| 10.17 | Minimize Stress | 104 |
| 10.18 | What were you put on this Earth for? | 105 |

# About the Author

Janice wrote this book so that you can understand how your body works and better take care of yourself and know that the possibilities are immense for slowing down the ageing process and boosting up the feel good factor in your life. Janice is that health consultant who will tell you the root cause of what is going on with your health and help you fix it. Janice also gives talks about health to inspire people to do better. From someone who wanted to know how to hold back the years and feel good, to actually finding out, at great financial expense, but what would have been the cost otherwise? Immeasurable!

Janice believes there is no cost greater than not knowing how to treat yourself well and she wants everyone to be able to do just that.

# Foreword

The Keys to Your Health is a book that will make you think and question everything you have been told about what is healthy with a critical eye and give you the incentive to do your own research and due diligence with your proper glasses on. These glasses will help you to look at your body and the way it is supposed to work in nature and compare it with what we are doing to it in this modern world and decipher which is the correct path. The knowledge in this book will truly help you to take your energy to another level.

# Acknowledgments

I express my deep appreciation for Derin Bepo whom, without him, this book would not be possible at all. He taught me so much and led me down this path of health excellence. Peter Pure is also a great contributor to my health knowledge, I can't thank them both enough. You both built on the knowledge I acquired from the British School of Osteopathy. From the bottom of my heart I want to thank Sharon Smith without whom I would know nothing about Vishal Morjaria or the WOW book camp, who taught me how to write this book and get it published in quick time. Sharon's tireless responses to my questions whenever I asked her for her opinion on this fact or that statement, and I asked a lot, really helped. A huge thanks to Vivienne Williams my close friend who supported me as only she could and Ritzy who gave me really useful advice about how to focus and get the job done. I also take the time for all the readers who trust me enough to buy this book and use the information to their best ability.

# Note to the reader

This book is designed to provide accurate information in regard to the subject matter covered. It is sold with the understanding that the publisher is not engaged in giving medical advice or services and that without personal consultation the author cannot give any advice or judgement about a particular patient or condition. While every attempt has been made to provide accurate information, the publisher and author cannot be held responsible for any errors or omissions. The final decision to engage in any treatment should be made together with you and your primary care consultant.

# CHAPTER 1
# Define What Health Is

### Healthy at 90

Is health more than just the absence of disease? Ask yourself this question. If you have no chronic illness to speak of but you struggle to sleep, you have lost your appetite, your skin has got a grey pallor to it or you have no energy but you have a clean bill of health from your doctor, you must be ok. Does that mean you are healthy? What about your emotional health or a negative mind set? Are you still healthy?

Health, in my book, is when you are vital, full of energy, and you feel like you could jump over the roof. You know you are at the top of your game when you are happy and you feel on top of the world all without the need for any drugs. My health is my wealth.

People have low expectations when it comes to being healthy and as you get into your senior years, like 60 and beyond, or even 50, people think that it's only natural that, as you get older, you get the common old age diseases. Arthritis, high blood pressure, middle age spread, having less energy, starting to lose your eyesight or developing dementia are accepted as normal.

## Old age doesn't mean unhealthy

I don't want to be normal. I don't want to be mediocre. Ill health and old age do not have to go hand in hand at all, it all depends on how you live. It does not depend only on your genes. You have the genes that you received from your fore parents but it's your lifestyle that determines if those genes are expressed or not. You might have the gene that makes you more vulnerable to getting diabetes but it's your lifestyle that turns the genes on or off and that determines whether diabetes is expressed or not.

## Epigenetics

There is a term called epigenetics, which means above the gene. You may have the gene for prostate cancer but it does not appear, because you used what is known as epigenetic actions which turned off the gene for prostate cancer so you never get it. All you do is live a life that protects you against the cancer and makes it very difficult for cancer to get a hold. All that really means is keeping a strong immune system by living in a healthy way.

Having your breasts cut off because you have the BRC 2

gene and you are scared of getting breast cancer is an action that comes out of not having all the information. You are in control of your health destiny. There is little need to fear these degenerative diseases when you know how to slow down the ageing process and look after yourself properly. We have the genetic potential to live until we are 120 years old and still be in good health. Most people spend the last 10 to 20 years of their lives being chronically ill and life is not supposed to be that way. We are supposed to only get sick or tired just 2 or 3 months before we die, or even less than that when our body is worn out and can no longer sustain us.

## The way we live makes a difference

Take two Ford Capri cars that were manufactured at the same time and they are the same model so they are exactly the same age and one of them is owned by a very careful driver who drives it for half an hour every day and keeps it locked up in a garage. The other one is owned by a travelling salesman who clocked up 50,000 miles a year on the clock. Which one do you think would be in better nick after 10 years? I would guess the one that is kept in the garage and we, as humans, are the same. We are mechanical so if we look after ourselves really, really well, we last longer and have better health.

## Inflammatory foods cause problems

Inflammation is the basis of all chronic diseases and inflammation is our body's defence against toxins and microbes so it is a good thing but we don't want to be inflamed all the time because that is when we age quickly and succumb to the diseases that we are oh so familiar with. Certain foods cause damage and therefore we could have inflammation inside our bodies without us realising. They call it silent inflammation, when you can't feel the symptoms of the cells response to try and clear up the damage. We keep on eating the inflammatory food and keep stoking the fire of inflammation so that it does not go away and it becomes chronic. Chronic is the same as long term. If you carry on with the actions that cause inflammation, it will eventually kill you. Look at any health issues we have; psoriasis, haemorrhoids, multiple sclerosis etc. and you will find inflammation from some damage that we are inadvertently causing to ourselves. We can consume foods that are anti-inflammatory that put out the fire and make us feel better, by reducing pain, reducing brain fog, reducing allergies and autoimmune diseases. Many of these problems are caused by ignorance and being told misinformation so we think we are doing the right thing and we are doing absolutely the opposite.

Nobody is the same, we are all so different and some of us can eat the healthiest diet and still get sick. That is not because they are eating the wrong food but because their system is not in an optimum state to handle it. If you cannot handle the most basic, easy to absorb food, and that would be the food that has the highest water content, then there is something seriously wrong with your guts. Antibiotics are just one of the time bombs that can decimate your ability to break down simple foods and make it easier for you to process junk food, making you reluctant to eat well. I will talk in more detail about that in another chapter.

## Drugs cause epigenetic diseases

What do I mean by that? You may not necessarily have the genes for Alzheimer's, but you get it anyway because you are taking high blood pressure medication and the side effect is Alzheimer's. All drugs have side effects. Every single drug, including Aspirin, has side effects and will block your pathways and destroy your enzymes, so they may cause diseases that you may not even have the genes for. That is epigenetics; where you do something that is above the gene, causing a disease to occur. Or it can prevent and cure diseases.

ACE inhibitors, given for heart disease, cause zinc deficiencies and zinc is essential for muscle function and sphincter and valve control. The heart is a muscle and needs zinc to be strong, so can you see the paradox.

Beta blockers are given for heart disease and they deplete Co-enzyme Q10, an enzyme that puts energy in the muscles. The heart is a muscle that needs energy so what do you think will happen after that? Beta blockers also deplete melatonin which is necessary for getting a good night's sleep and melatonin also protects against cancer, so you might need to take sleeping pills along with your beta blockers.

Statins, cholesterol lowering drugs, can cause dementia, diabetes, difficulties digesting fats, reduce Vitamin D and weaken muscles amongst other things. In the United States they know that statins deplete Co-enzyme Q10 (which is crucial for your heart energy) so they give you Co-enzyme Q10 every time they give you statins because they are afraid of being sued. In the UK they don't do that.

Proton pump inhibitors (PPI's), given when you have acid reflux to solve the risk of adenocarcinomas, actually cause adenocarcinomas, oesophageal cancer. When PPI's were first brought to the market, it was recommended that they be used short term; no longer than 3 to 6 weeks. People stay on these drugs for years and they cause osteoporosis because they stop the absorption of calcium and many other minerals. You cannot absorb your nutrients properly if you don't have the correct level of acids. If they were working you would get better quickly and you would not need to take them anymore. Nobody is looking at the bigger picture, to find the root cause and giving the solution but Gaviston is one of the biggest money makers for the big pharmaceutical industry.

Anti-depressants taken long term can cause depression. There are many other drugs that cause chronic diseases. Drugs are never the answer because your body always does the right thing, you just need to trust it. If you have a symptom, you should really be asking yourself what went wrong, or what have I done or what have I been eating and how can I reverse it?

Most drugs actually cause the very problem that they are supposed to solve.

## The organs work in sync

The body works as a whole. All the organs work in sync with each other. The kidney does not work separately from the heart or the liver. If one is having problems it will have a knock on effect on the other organs but when we get treated with conventional medicine they will look at everything separately as if they are independent, stand-a-lone organs that have no effect on the rest of the body.

## Your body is always talking to you

Listen to your body because when you get a symptom, it is telling you something. It is trying to get your attention. You don't have migraines because you are short of co-codamol or the preferred drug of the day. You have migraines because your body is reacting to something it might be short of, like water or reacting to something that it doesn't like. Maybe drugs can be good for a short term problem but at the end of the day, you really want to find out what is causing the problem so that you can sort it out and get back to balance.

If you have to take a drug for months or years to suppress symptoms, you will never be well because drugs are not the answer. To be healthy you need to regenerate cells and you are not going to regenerate with drugs.

Degeneration and ageing are two separate things and arthritis, dementia, diabetes, obesity and other diseases are degeneration. Ageing is just you getting older but you don't have to get sicker. There is no need to fear old age when you know what to do and that is truly what ageing gracefully is all about.

# CHAPTER 2
# Water

### Water is life

Water is crucial to being a healthy human so discovering the best water that will increase your longevity is worth putting some thought into. Our body's water levels are the same as the planet Earth and what benefits the planet also benefits us, meaning we need to keep our bodies pristine and free from chemicals.

Metabolic processes, of which there are thousands every second going on in our body, cannot be carried out without water. Water is the best solute there is and that allows our cells to use the nutrients and minerals in the biological processes. Processes like energy being created in the cell needs water. We have cells like batteries where the energy we need to do everything is produced. Regulating our temperature needs water. Food absorption in our intestines needs water. Minerals and vitamins crossing membranes and hormones travelling in our blood all need water in order to do their job. The human being consists of about 75% water and as we age that reduces to about 60%. So if our bodies are made with such a large percentage of water, it only makes sense that we need to be drinking the best and the purest water we can find.

## Dehydration dangers

Dehydration of our cells damages the kidneys. Imagine you are looking at a pond that has dried up and there is only mud at the bottom and there are fish in there that are flapping about in the mud trying not to die. Kidneys filter about 200 litres of fluid every day, so if they cannot do their job properly because of dehydration, they would be like the fish in that pond. Toxins would build up in the body, causing kidney failure and can cause symptoms like high blood pressure, headaches, fluid retention as your body tries to hold on to as much liquid as it can, headaches, lower back pain and more. When you get a headache the last thing most of us think is "I probably need more water". Dehydration is a factor in many diseases.

Water; try living without it and you won't last much longer than a week. In order to maintain our levels of water to the most optimum, we need to be replacing all the water that we lose via breathing, sweating, defecating, urinating and vomiting. Adults lose about two pints of water at night when we sleep, through the skin and by breathing. The first thing we should do when we get up is to drink water and replace what we have lost. But not just any old water.

## What water should we drink?

What is the best water that we should be drinking? Structured water is the best and that is normally structured by plants, for example, coconut water straight out of a fresh green coconut because coconut water has minerals and vitamins that are so similar to the plasma in human blood that it has been known to be used in blood transfusions during the Second World War when plasma was in short supply. Coconut water is a naturally structured water and filtered by the tree that has been soaking up the minerals from the soil and the water under the ground and it is alive. It is full of all the important electrolytes like magnesium, calcium, potassium, and sodium. The minerals have the proper charge for our body to absorb more fully. Coconut water has antioxidants that will counteract ageing and help us stay free of disease.

Green juice is another excellent type of structured water and if you really want to take control of your health and feel better right away, there is nothing better than a green juice made from vegetables full of vitamins, minerals and nutrients for life. These are the molecules that build your bodies system so that it can function at its best. Taking the juice out of the plant makes it easier to be absorbed by the body and it gives you a quick hit of healing power from the raw enzymes. Enzymes are proteins that direct the life force into your metabolic processes and help to repair your DNA. Green juice helps to detoxify, cleanse and alkalize your system and is an excellent source of calcium and iron. Where do you think the large vegetarian animals get their calcium and iron from, like the cow, the horse, the hippopotamus and the giraffe? They aren't drinking any cow's milk or eating any cheese.

## Machines that treat water

There are many machines that do amazing things with water. We have alkalizers, distillers, reverse osmosis filters, vortex magnetisers, and water restructurers. They all have their unique ways of making water better. We even have water softening equipment but I would not recommend them for drinking. In fact, the installers will tell you that you can't drink the water so you end up having to buy water for drinking and cooking.

Alkalizing machines are also ionizers and they claim to raise the pH of drinking water by using electrolysis to separate the water stream into acidic and alkaline streams. The acid portion can be used to clean surfaces. The alkaline portion helps to neutralize the acidity coming from an acid diet but it needs to be drunk straight from the machine because it only lasts for 24 hours, after that it is not effective anymore. Alkalizing machines are also known to triple the antioxidant potential of vitamins C.

Distillers and reverse osmosis machines are the most thorough at getting rid of solutes in the water and will eradicate 99% of them but they leave your water lacking in natural minerals and you would do best to add some minerals back in.

Vortex magnetized water is said to structure and vitalize your water to make it taste better, move more freely into the cell, and make it more difficult for toxins to build up in the body so it is better for detoxifying, has a superior energy flow and is healthier for drinking.

Some machines are said to restructure your water without vortexing and they make the molecule size of the water smaller, making it more wet, which makes it more absorbable by the body. It seems there is more to water than just H2O. The structure of water is more important than its chemical composition. The structure is how its molecules are organised. Water molecules join together into groups called clusters and it's the smaller cluster size that makes getting into the cells much easier.

## No to tap water

Tap water seems to be the worst kind of water there is because it has additives, chemicals, chlorine, fluoride and microbes and they don't taste very nice. Filtering water is a must these days and if you do not use a filter then you become the filter. Look inside a kettle and see the build-up of gunk over time, well that is what is building up in your system, possibly causing blockages of arteries, kidneys, calcification and stiffness in soft tissue in your brain, breast, lungs, eyes, joints, or wherever your weak link is. So because you feel ok at the moment, it is better to think long term and try to avoid any possible problems in the future.

## We don't want plastic water

Bottled water is a big problem, not only because it is kept in plastic bottles which leach into the water, but also because these plastic bottles are ending up in the sea and choking our sea creatures and we end up eating the plastic in those fish so it all comes around full circle. The longer the water stands in the plastic bottle in the supermarket and the warmer the temperature gets, the more plastic you will end up drinking and plastic (made from petroleum) is an endocrine disruptor. Spring bottled water has very few regulations so you might find toxins in there that you don't want to drink, like arsenic for example. A lot of the bottled water comes straight from the tap and they just filter it and put a label on it called spring water so it is very hard to know which water you can trust.

## We definitely need a filter

Carbon block filters are useful because you can get a whole house carbon block filter which can filter out the chlorine in your shower, bathroom, and washing machine and everywhere in your house so you don't have to worry at all.

Choose which machine is the best one for your needs but whatever you do, do not drink tap water without a filter.

# CHAPTER 3
# The Micro Biome

### Health starts with the gut

Why the gut, because the gut feeds everything. The food comes into the gut, gets mixed with digestive juices, and then it goes into the intestines where more juices are mixed in and it is churned up a little more and it travels into the blood stream and out to every cell in the body. In other words, the gut feeds everything. Your brain needs proper nutrition so imagine if it doesn't get it, perhaps ADHD or Alzheimer's or depression could be the result. Your joints need nutrition so if they don't get what they need arthritis will result. Bones need nutrition too and without it you get osteoporosis.

Imagine if what you feed your gut was poisonous to your system. Then you could get sick or even worse; die. It is crucial to feed your system a healthy diet in order to have healthy cells in order to be a healthy you. What you feed your body today becomes your cells of tomorrow.

The micro biome is the foundation of staying in good shape so when you learn how to look after it and keep it in the best condition you will not only survive but you will thrive and that is what I am going to teach you in this book.

You have a few of these micro biomes throughout your body, the biggest and most important one being in your gut. You also have one on your skin, in your mouth, nasal passage, eyes, urinary tract and more.

## Micro biome: What is it?

It is one of the hottest topics in medical research today. The micro biome is a community of microbes consisting of bacteria, viruses, protozoa, and prions that work together like a community to do the job of protecting you against infection, keeping your mucous membranes healthy, making hormones, and making vitamins. In the gut, it also makes neurotransmitters, alters your pH, affects your inflammatory responses and breaks down your food because without it you cannot assimilate your nutrients. The micro biome is responsible for the way you think, your mood, your hormonal balance, bone strength, your immune system and many other things. Gut health determines the health of the human. Your gut, together with your liver, comprise 80% of your immune system. Everybody has a unique micro biome just like everybody has unique finger prints and the reason for that is that the gut responds to the environment and no two environments can be exactly the same.

## Where do we get our microbes from?

We get our microbes originally from our mother's birth canal. The mother can only give you what she has got so the more diversity she has, the better, but if you are born via C section, you will have a totally different micro biome than if you were born via the birth canal and you will have less microbes. As we experience life we interact with more varied microbes from everything we touch. A baby that is breast fed will have different microbes than a baby fed on formula and the longer you are breast fed the more changes the microbes make. Antibiotics can have a devastating effect on children for years and even for life without anyone connecting the dots. You will just be seen as a sickly baby and you could have allergies and auto immune diseases as well due to the immune system being compromised. A fever can shift your micro biome, especially if you try to stop the body from doing what it does best, because a fever is generally what the body does deliberately to kill the microbes by overheating them. Stress, injury, and change in diet all change the biome. Pregnancy changes the flora of the canal getting ready for the baby. Puberty and menopause will also have an effect. Gender, climate, your career, how clean you are and even our genes effect the micro biome population by changing the acidity of the gut.

Fluoride, chlorine in the water, processed foods, pesticides, agrochemicals, GMO's, pills, vaccines, chemicals all have a negative effect on our microbes. It reflects everything we have done in our lives and everywhere we have been. When we use harsh abrasives on our skin or anti-bacterial wipes we are destroying the microbes that protect our skin against diseases like psoriasis and eczema.

## Does it all boil down to your genes?

The cells in your gut outnumber the cells in your body by 10 to one. Imagine having 10 times more bacteria than we have cells and then imagine each of those bacteria having numerous genes of their own. That is a whole lot of genes so when people talk about genetics affecting our health they should really be considering the genetics belonging to our micro biome.

Why do some people feel sick at the site of a cucumber or heave at the smell of mint and other people are okay with them? What if the reason is because we don't have the bacteria to break those foods down and our body is reacting because we would struggle if we tried to eat them? Every time you eat, you are feeding your micro biome. When you eat apples you are feeding the apple digesting microbes and when you eat bread you are feeding the wheat and yeast digesting microbes. Every time you feed any particular microbes they increase in number. When we are told to eat a wide variety of food that is the reason why, so that we are feeding a large variety of microbes and they will be able to break down anything and everything. We need a balance.

You could say that your gut starts at the mouth and goes all the way to the anus because we are a tube that is open to the elements. Good bacteria lining the whole of the gastro intestinal tract will ensure that there is no room for any harmful bacteria to lodge and cause problems because all the spaces are already taken so the harmful bacteria will just go straight through the body and out the other side without causing any harm.

## Three billion bacteria are shared from the mouth to the gut every day

You can quite clearly see how 80% of chronic diseases start with problems in the mouth. Streptococcus is a bacteria that causes strep throat and once it enters the blood stream it can cause permanent damage to the heart valves. Mercury in the mouth, known as silver fillings, are toxic to the nerves. It is the second most toxic element on the planet after plutonium and they put it in our teeth right next to our brains. People have been known to suffer from severe migraines all their life and as soon as they take the toxic mercury from their teeth their migraine goes away. Heavy metals have a detrimental effect on your gut health because it will reduce the amount of good bacteria you have. We want to keep a clean mouth and that also means not having any root canals because all root canals are infected and weaken our immune system. There is no way that the thousands and thousands of little tubules that run perpendicular to the main canal can be cleaned and they can destroy your enzymes when they are toxic. Just to show how serious a root canal is, Doctor Hal Huggins, after 23 years of dental practice, said he had never found a breast cancer patient who did not have a root canal treatment or a cavity in the bicuspid -meridian. All teeth have a meridian running through them that connects to another part of the body. Doctor. Blanche Grube, a biological dentist, said that she could not read all the way through school, despite taking extra reading lessons. In college she still couldn't read. She had one mercury filling removed and the next day she could read.

### Stress affects your micro biome

Stress is the biggest killer and that is because it affects your hormones which affect your micro biome. The stress hormone is cortisol and when it comes out it suppresses the activity of your gut because if you are seriously stressed, your body thinks it's running away from some kind of threat. The most important thing in that moment is to get out of there, so cortisol will help you to do that by fuelling your muscles with enough energy to run from the danger, or perceived danger. Digestion is not needed at this time so it is shut down and it stops working, causing bloating or wind later on. Your immune system is unnecessary as well and that is suppressed making you vulnerable to diseases. High cortisol levels over a long period of time consistently put energy, such as glucose, into your blood (energy comes from the breakdown of the muscle) causing chronic high sugar levels leading to skinny arms and legs, round body, diabetes, and adrenal fatigue. Cortisol also suppresses insulin production because insulin is the fat storing hormone and right now you want to use the energy to run from the threat and not store it as fat. Cortisol causes insulin resistance, which makes you more vulnerable to getting Type II diabetes. As soon as the stressor has gone what happens to all that sugar in the blood? It then gets stored as fat and that is why you can gain the weight.

The adrenal glands are where the cortisol and adrenalin comes from and if you are producing them constantly the adrenal glands will get tired and fatigued, especially if they are not supported by adequate nutrition.

### The gut connection to Alzheimer's

The gut plays an important role in Alzheimer's because you can eat your way into Alzheimer's and you can also reverse it if it is not too advanced. Trans-fats and sugars are not good for your brain. Sugars also incorporate carbohydrates like potato, grain, and starches because they turn to sugar very quickly in the body before it hits your stomach. For example, bread, pizza, chips, biscuits, cakes and anything made from flour will turn to sugar. The problem with eating sugar is that it binds with protein, the two nutrients together form glycation-end products, which is very ageing, especially for the skin, and causes those degenerative diseases previously discussed. Alzheimer's patients have a lot of a substance called amyloid plaque in the brain. Amyloid plaque is formed by glycation. It is very sticky and it forms a barrier between the brain's nerve cells so that they cannot communicate with each other properly, reducing memory. This amyloid plaque builds up over time and you see the situation getting slowly worse.

## Brains are made of saturated fat

Fat is very good for your brain because your brain is made of mostly saturated fat. If you eat low fat or unsaturated fats you will be robbing your brain of the very raw material it needs to function optimally. Quality is what's important when it comes to feeding your brain. Trans-fats are damaging not just to your brain but to every cell in your body because they are not recognised by the body as food. The body just has to deal with them the best it can. What are trans-fats? Trans-fats are created when you cook any fat because you change the molecular structure of the fat to something totally different. Hydrogenated fat is very unhealthy and is formed when a fat that is normally soft at room temperature, like an oil, has hydrogen bonds forced into the molecule in order to turn it into a solid fat. So now it's a fat that is solid at room temperature, like they do with margarine. Margarine is one molecule away from plastic, which is why it is so damaging to the body; it is so unnatural.

## The role of the gut in colitis

Colitis is inflammation of the colon. Not everyone suffers from this but what separates those who have it from those who do not? Good question. Two people of the same age, sex, job, stress levels, eating exactly the same food could have different outcomes. One could get colitis and the other gets nothing. It all depends on your micro biome.

Feeding your gut substances that cause inflammation time and time again will initially feel okay and you may not notice that there is a problem but after a time the body can't make up for it anymore and colitis, IBS and other gut problems could result. It all depends on what your weakest link is. The most likely culprit that causes problems with the gut are grains like wheat, barley and rye because they contain gluten. It does not matter if you are eating bread and it's organic or three seeded because it's still gluten and gluten is the problem. Dairy is also another huge problem for a lot of people but, really, if you are eating junk then you should not be surprised if you get into trouble.

## Faecal transplants work

Faecal transplant is a treatment that has been used for hundreds of years and even used in veterinary medicine, yet

I have only recently heard of it. I have heard how miraculous it can be for treating dogs as well as humans. It comprises of using the faeces of one human and transplanting it into the colon of another human who is sick in order to change their micro biome for the better. This is done by using capsules that are swallowed or suppositories in the anus. You might find that once is not enough and generally you have to do this a few times. It can turn you around from deaths door to bright and breezy in no time.

### Xenoestrogen's can cause breast cancer

Breast cancer is very common these days and most of them are hormone driven. Oestrogen is the hormone that drives it. The source of most of the oestrogen is from xenoestrogens, which are endocrine disruptors derived from chemicals, they are not a natural hormone but they mimic the real thing in the body. When you slap on that make-up or perfume or moisturizer that contains so many different chemicals that you can't even pronounce their names, give a thought for what effect it has on your biggest organ, your skin. Cleaning liquids, that shower gel, surface cleaner or disinfectant all get on your skin, into your blood stream and into your guts and effects your micro biome in a bad way.

## You are in control of your micro biome

How you can influence your micro biome. Every time you eat, you are feeding your micro biome so we just need to make sure we are in balance. If you eat junk food all day you will be feeding your bad bacteria and they will be proliferating and overtaking. The same is also true for the good bacteria. Ultimately you are in the driver's seat and it is all within your own control. Putting your bare hands in the soil will increase your bio diversity in the gut so getting an allotment or doing some gardening, if you are lucky enough to have a garden, will be a huge benefit to your health. Being connected to the earth also has some fantastic benefits. Check out Clint Ober's "Earthing: The Most Important Discovery Ever". Also, any drugs, recreational or otherwise, will have a devastating effect on our guts.

# CHAPTER 4

# Are We Designed To Eat meat?

**What are we designed to eat?**

There are so many diets out there. We have the vegetarian diet, the vegan diet, the omnivore diet, the paleo diet, the ketogenic diet, and Weight Watchers. Which one is the right one for us or are they all okay in moderation.

What we used to eat in the past doesn't mean that we should be eating it now. What do you think someone in 1000 years' time, who looks back at the way we eat today, will think about today's diet? Do you think they will say to themselves, yes they ate this and they ate that, so that obviously means that we should be eating the same? What we have eaten in the past has no bearing on what we are designed to eat, because we eat loads of food that is inadvertently killing us.

Carnivorous animals can eat cereals, because that is what kibble is, but that doesn't mean they should be eating it. Why do you think true carnivores, like cats, get diabetes? We are feeding them a diet that they are not designed to eat.

Look at the lifespan of the Eskimo's and look at what they eat. They live on average about 10 years less than the rest of the Canadian population. Eskimo's also look very old due to their leathery looking skin.

Look at the blue zones where there are a lot of centenarians. What do they eat? The longest lived group of people in America are the Seventh Day Adventist's who are pushed forward as an example of how to live a longer and a healthier life and check out what they eat.

## Gathering the evidence

Look at any living thing and you will see that all beings have to be able to procure their food in an energy efficient manner because if you spend more energy getting and absorbing your food than you get from eating your food then you will not survive for long. Everything living is given the equipment needed to be able to efficiently get the food they need to survive, even through pregnancy.

Let's look at the evidence. What equipment have we been given that points to us being carnivorous or herbivorous? We have to look at our anatomy and physiology to see if we can find clues. How would we survive with the equipment we have been given? Some people are going to say we have been given a brain to think so that we can use it to manufacture equipment that we can use to capture and kill animals that we might not otherwise have access to. I'm not thinking about that,

I am only thinking about the equipment we have from birth. What kind of equipment are we born with?

Carnivores eat other animals that don't want to be eaten so they will run away and as a carnivore you have to be fast enough to catch them. You need the teeth that can bring down, kill and consume an animal; hoofs, hair, bones and all. Carnivores will always go for the weaker animals like the old or the young or injured or sicker animals, because they are easier to catch and it also keeps the gene pool of the prey a lot stronger. We don't know whether that is on their mind when they are hunting but maybe that is just a beneficial side effect.

Herbivores have the problem of having to search and forage far and wide to gather enough food for them to eat and feel full, so they are always grazing. Herbivores are made for walking and are lousy runners so you can walk for long periods without using too much energy because walking is really a controlled falling. You just kick one leg out and fall forward and before you fall on your face the other leg has come forward and taken its place and this makes walking rather effortless. Herbivores seek out the prettiest, greenest and the best foliage because it generally has higher nutrition but humans will eat the best and the strongest animals as well, because they bring an herbivore mentality to a carnivorous diet and weaken the gene pool and cause the animals to become extinct.

Carnivores are built for speed and you can tell this because their legs are permanently flexed, always on their toes, as if they are always ready to pounce or launch into a sprint if anything delicious happens to pass by. Dogs and cats, you will notice when they are not doing anything in particular like walking from the front room to the front door, will go and lie down. Keeping your legs permanently flexed takes a lot of energy because your muscles are continually engaged. Carnivores are well padded and protected at the front of their body to reduce any injuries when the animal they are hunting kicks backwards. They have all their important organs right at the back where they are difficult to get injured and their weapons are right at the front.

There are two groups of herbivores, the ones that are hunted by the carnivores and the herbivores who are not hunted. The hunted group have very straight and slim, light weight limbs like the horse, the gazelle, and the dear compared to their body. These creatures do not use muscle power to stand up because it is the skeleton that keeps them upright. They use such a little amount of energy to stand up that they could easily fall asleep on their feet and they do. The herbivores that are not hunted, like the elephant, have straight, thick limbs because they don't need to run away since it's very rare for them to be hunted due to their size. The herbivores have a flat foot stance with their heel on the ground which is also called a plantigrade stance. Human beings are designed for walking, we have a plantigrade stance.

The vulnerable parts of our anatomy are way up front where it is very easy for them to get damaged by prey and predators are not normally designed that way. Most predators are usually asleep during the day and as human beings our night vision is so terrible because we are designed to be awake during the day and to sleep at night.

Every female of every species is designed to be able to get the food she needs, even when pregnant, to survive. Heavily pregnant humans are not good at hunting and herbivores have much longer pregnancies and they tend to have one baby at a time. Carnivorous female animals have a short pregnancy, less than 3 months long, so that they can carry on hunting without too much interference. Predators have litters and they are born at a much younger age than herbivores and the typical baby weight is less than 3% of the mother's body weight. Herbivore babies are generally 7 to 8% of the mother's body weight.

Let's have a look at the head of a carnivore where the teeth are designed for cutting and ripping.

You don't have to season up a piece of meat and cook it to make a lion want to eat it. If humans are really designed to eat it we would be salivating and smacking our lips when we see a living animal. The diet that we are currently eating is the cause of 80% of the heart disease and all we have to do is eat what we are designed to eat to reverse most of the modern day diseases. Would you put lemonade into a car engine and expect it to run efficiently? That is essentially what we are doing with our bodies when we eat inappropriate foods and then we say "why me" when we get sick.

Our physiology determines our diet. Let's compare our anatomical and physiological differences to the animals and see where we fit in.

Carnivores want to eat other animals and the other animals want to run away so to be able to catch your food you have to be able to run fast and have teeth that can bring down your prey and kill it then tear the meat off the bone before it becomes cold and before it's been chopped up by a butcher and have no problems digesting every last morsel.

Herbivores, on the other hand, eat plants that don't run away so they are lousy runners but they are really efficient walkers and foragers. The plant food tends to be spread far and wide so they need to be designed for a lot of effortless walking to get enough food to eat.

Herbivores can suck water into their mouth by creating a vacuum in their mouth and carnivores can only lap up water.

## Who told you they were canines?

Look at the teeth of the carnivores, their canines are 3 times longer than their other teeth for piercing and tearing meat off the bone, they have molars that are sharp with jagged edges for cutting and shearing and herbivore molars have a flat surface for grinding because plant fibre is very tough.

Herbivores have spade like incisors for cropping and peeling plants. Our canines are so reduced in size that they function as accessory incisors. Herbivores can also move their jaws in a horizontal plane from side to side and carnivores can only move their jaws wide open and shut. The oesophagus (that is the tube that reaches from the throat to the stomach) is long, muscular and narrow because we can only take in small amounts of food at a time. Carnivores have a very short and wide oesophagus to enable them to get large quantities of food into their stomach at a time. Most people who choke to death every year, actually choke to death on meat.

The stomach of carnivores is also much larger than a herbivore's because they don't eat every day and they literally don't know when or where their next meal is coming from so when they do manage to catch some prey they will eat till they are full and they can consume about 30%-40% of their body weight. Try eating 30% of your body weight in one go and see if you can. For a 60kg human that would be about 20kg of food.

Carnivores are designed for intermittent fasting which means maybe eating once a week because when you are a hunter you just don't eat every day. Even humans in the ancient civilizations when the men went to hunt the meat and bring it back to the village would not eat meat every day but they obviously had other things to eat on a daily basis apart from meat. Humans are designed to eat at least once a day.

High oxidized cholesterol causes heart disease and stroke

in humans. We cannot adequately break down the protein and fat contained in animal flesh. Meat has no fibre and at any one time humans have about 12 pounds of undigested putrefying meat lodged in their intestines. Dogs and cats cannot get high cholesterol because their liver produces really strong bile that will break down the fat far more efficiently than our bile does. For that same reason they don't get gall stones either. Their stomach acid is a lot lower than ours, and that is needed to be able to break down the bone, feathers, hoofs, hair, the offal and all the muscle meat that comes from their prey. If our stomach acid was that low we would not be able to survive.

After the food leaves the stomach carnivores have a very short intestine because the food is so acidic that it needs to be removed as soon as possible. The intestines are 3 to 6 times longer than the body of the animal and the enzymes in the small intestine are predominately for breaking down fat and protein. It is not easy for them to digest a lot of carbohydrates. The body is measured from the top of the head to the top of the tail. Carnivores do not chew their food. There is no point because they do not have any enzymes in the mouth to start the breakdown of the carbohydrates like humans have and the whole point of chewing is to mix the food with the enzymes and only plant eaters have that. All carnivores want to do is get the food into the stomach where the acid can start digestion. Human intestines are long and winding because of the fibre in our food and it takes a lot of work to get the nutrients out of the food because the plant fibre is tough and cannot be broken down completely but it does the job of keeping the intestines clean and feeding the micro biome. Our intestines are 10 to12 times longer than our body. Only plant eaters have an appendix. Herbivores cannot detoxify vitamin A but carnivores can. Herbivores can make vitamin A from beta carotene but carnivores cannot.

Let's look at the colon of the carnivores. They have short and smooth colons which is only designed for elimination because by the time waste gets to the colon it has no nutrition in it and it needs to come out before it starts to putrefy and release toxins. Herbivores have a colon that is long and pouched because there is still work to be done, vitamins to be made, fermentation of more of the fibre and absorption of liquid from out of the faeces.

Eating animal flesh is not just about opening your mouth and putting it in because many people are becoming more aware of what goes into bringing that animal to your plate and why vegetarianism and veganism is growing in the west because factory animal farms produce meat through routine torture and environmental destruction. Little consideration is given to the animal or the consumer. They are treated like things and not like beings with their own personality and wants and needs. For example none of them want to die and they are raised in such dirty environments that they use up 80% of the antibiotics that are made and only 20% goes for human health. These animals are tortured both mentally and physically because of their confinement where they don't have the space to turn around and it drives them literally mad. Adrenaline is high in these confined animal feeding operations and you can smell the fear. When we eat these creatures we get all that angst, all that adrenaline, all the antibiotics (this could be why antibiotic resistant diseases are on the rise), all the GMO feed that they are given, pesticide laden grains and hormones. We get it all, not to mention the second rate protein and inferior fat.

To conclude human beings who stick closely to the herbivores diet are more likely to have an ideal weight, be the longest lived and when we stray from that ideal we get very sick. We are so used to being omnivores but at the same time we are so used to being sick. The human body does best as an herbivore.

# CHAPTER 5
# Sleep

### What is the point of sleep?

Good quality sleep is extremely important if you want to have optimal health because our cells need to rest, repair and rejuvenate so that you wake up in the morning feeling younger than you went to bed. Sleep will also clean out the system, from 4am -12pm midday, our body is cleaning out all the organs and cells. The glial cells in the brain maintain the brain neurons and keep them clean and nourished and makes new brain cells, which helps memory and function. Have you ever gone to bed thinking about a problem that you don't know the answer to and when you wake up in the morning you think of the solution straight away? Well that is because our brain has been cleaned overnight and now it is more efficient.

Sleep is actually just as important as eating good quality food because exhaustion from lack of sleep can make us sleepy during the day, slow to react to situations, have memory loss, slow to process information, make bad decisions, compromise performance and it will age you quicker. Every cell in your body will be aged, not just your skin. You can eat the best food, think the best thoughts, drink the best water and breath the best air but if you can't sleep, everything else has little benefit. Shortage of certain minerals, vitamins and hormones will scupper a good night's sleep. The most important mineral is melatonin and you can't get melatonin without serotonin and you can't get serotonin without tryptophan and you can't get tryptophan without eating the right diet. Almost all serotonin and tryptophan are made in the digestive tract and only a small amount in the brain.

**Insomnia can cause diabetes**

Sleep deprivation will alter your hormones, because lack of sleep is stressful to the body and will cause cortisol, the stress hormone, to rise, suppressing the immune system, dumping sugar into the blood, interfering with digestion and making you wired and tired. Cortisol has its own natural time to release and decrease in the body and is in rhythm with the master clock through the adrenal glands. Leptin is the hormone that tells your stomach when it is full and satisfied. Ghrelin tells your body when it is hungry. Both these hormones are disturbed with lack of sleep to the extent that leptin is reduced so that you never feel full and Ghrelin is increased so you always feel hungry and that is how sleeplessness can contribute to obesity and diabetes.

## How much sleep is enough sleep?

That depends on how much growth and regeneration is going on because at both ends of the scale sleep needs are very different. Babies sleep a lot more because they are growing a lot. Elders need less sleep usually because their cell turnover has slowed right down so there is not much repair and regeneration going on. For the people in between, it depends on how active you are. If you play hard and work hard during the day you will need to sleep hard to get that repair, so athletes will probably need more sleep than the average person. When people are mentally unwell (depressed or have OCD) they tend to sleep quite a lot or can't sleep at all because their master clock has been disrupted. Sleep deprivation is as bad for your immune system as stress or disease, which explains why night shift workers have higher rates of cancer, heart disease and all the chronic diseases. Sleep deprivation is so detrimental that it was used in the 2nd World War in the concentration camps as a torture and is one of the quickest ways to break a man's spirit, both mentally and physically. Let me explain.

## How lack of sleep causes disease

All creatures need to be in tune with the rhythm of the planet, it's called your circadian rhythm or your internal 24hr clock that is always running in the background. The tide comes in and out at the same time every day. The sun rises and falls every day. These things are dead certain and happen without fail year after year century after century. Every process in nature is orderly. We need to be in tune with that rhythm. Humans need to be sleeping when the sun goes down and rising when the sun rises because light sets our circadian rhythm, which is our master clock, the biological clock that is in our brain, and this clock sets all the other clocks in our body. The stomach, liver, kidney and the heart all contain hormone producing cells and glands that will be negatively affected when we are out of sync with our biological clock and can cause havoc with your thirst, hunger, sexual desire, body fat levels and lots of other functions. One hormone relies on another so it can cause a whole cascade of disruption. Once you understand how it works, it is very easy to understand how lack of sleep can lead to many chronic diseases.

## How we set our natural body clock

Exposure to natural light during the day helps you set your biological clock so that you sleep better at night, midday being the optimal time to get your exposure because that is when the sun is at its strongest. Day workers, who are exposed to unnatural light all day and finish work when it is dark, would benefit from a small amount, at least 20 minutes, of real sun exposure at lunchtime. Darkness at night is the other side of the equation that gets you to sleep. So strong light in the day and pitch blackness at night is what instigates your pineal gland to manufacture melatonin and melatonin is your sleep hormone, without which you cannot get to sleep. Melatonin also contains potent cancer fighting properties because it inhibits the acceleration of cancer cell growth and promotes apoptosis (cancer cell death).

## How to get beauty sleep

Digesting food is hard work for the body and uses up about 60% of its resources. Eating and drinking (especially if it's a stimulant like coffee or alcohol) late at night gives your body a heavy job to do so it cannot rest at the same time. You can never get rested sleep when you go to bed with a full stomach and it is THE most ageing thing you can do. The term beauty sleep is often quoted for a reason.

## Light is important for well being

In ancient times, before technology, people would sleep when the sun went down and wake when the sun rose. Today we have electricity so we can flick a switch and have light for 24 hours if we want to. This tells our brain that it is still daytime and confuses our master clock. Lights from computers, mobile phones, televisions etc. will also affect our inner clock but that is not all, because natural light in the day is predominantly blue and as the sun sets it becomes red triggering our sleep cycle. Our gadgets give off blue light so when we use them late at night we are giving mixed signals to our brain that it is time to be awake even though the timing says it's time to sleep. You can see how important light is to our wellbeing by observing the Icelandic population. In Iceland the longest day is about 21 hours of light and in the winter on the shortest day you get about 21 hours of darkness. The long, dark days are said to give a feeling of doom and gloom and has been blamed for the high depression rate in Iceland. One in ten people have depression, which is the fourth highest rate in Europe. On the other side of the coin, Icelanders are also said to be the happiest so they seem to flip from one extreme to the other.

## Electromagnetic radiation ionizes our cells

This disrupts our sleep. What is electromagnetic radiation? It is invisible energy that moves in waves, like radio waves, microwaves, x-rays and other waves. Smart meters, mobile phone masts and the base for the cordless phones give off very strong electromagnetic energy and when we are trying to sleep this is constantly bombarding our body making deep sleep very difficult. Baby monitors, Wi-Fi, pedometers, iPhones and iPads and other Wi-Fi devices are also damaging to the human physiology because not only are they using wireless technology but they emit blue light. It's not a good idea to have these devices in your bedroom when you are trying to sleep because it disturbs your pineal gland production of melatonin. Imagine living and sleeping in a microwave because that is what we are doing. 5G is the next generation of mobile phone technology that they are rolling out as we speak in 2017 and it will be one thousand times stronger than the 4G that we have already. This technology ionizes our cells. Ionizing radiation is dangerous because it puts calcium in the cell and damages the internal structure of the cell causing cell death and mutations. Insomnia is going to sky rocket, cancer is going to sky rocket and many chronic diseases will also sky rocket because this technology will surround the world like a blanket and there will be very few places to hide.

## Child night lights linked to depression

We are supposed to sleep in complete darkness and when mothers leave the lights on in the landing for their children because they are scared of the dark, they are causing so much harm. Child night lights have been linked to higher rates of obesity and depression because it disrupts the deep restorative sleep. During this deep restorative sleep, the human growth hormone is released to help with new cell growth and repair throughout the body, to strengthen our immune system and it also helps us manage our emotions.

## Deep sleep

How do you know when you have had enough sleep? If you wake up feeling tired then you probably didn't get enough deep restorative sleep. You cannot get back the sleep you have lost because once it's gone, it's gone. We are supposed to go through all the different stages of sleep. The deepest one being the most important so if we are continually interrupted, we can't get into the deep sleep. Remembering your dreams the day after is a sign that you slept deeply and you slept well. Being in bed for 8 hours and being continually interrupted so that you only get 4 hours of sleep has the same effect as having 4 hours in bed and only getting 4 hours sleep. Interrupted sleep has a cumulative affect and is just as damaging as lack of sleep and can be enormous. You should go through all 4 stages of sleep. Stage 1. You have decided to go to sleep and your eyes are closed but it is really easy to be woken up. Stage 2. Your bodily systems are starting to slow down in preparation for sleep. Stage 3. Brain waves slow down and you sleep through any potential sleep disturbances without any reaction and if you wake at this point you will be disoriented. Stage 4. Delta sleep, REM sleep, where the deepest most powerful dreams usually happen, your muscles are paralysed and this is where most people sleep walk or wet the bed.

## We need melatonin to sleep

We sleep in cycles of 60 to 90 minutes where we go through all four stages of sleep but not necessarily in numeric order and if your sleep gets disturbed, for example, by getting up to go to the toilet, you may not reach the deep restorative sleep state. If you do get up to go to the toilet, it is better if you don't turn on the light because that will signal your body that it is daytime and it's time to get up and you may struggle to get back to sleep. If you really struggle to navigate in the dark use a yellow, orange or red light because these colours do not shut down melatonin production in the same way as the white and blue bandwidth does. Most people think that getting up in the middle of the night is normal because everybody does it but it is not normal. When you are deep asleep, your bladder holds on until the morning because it doesn't feel the urges.

The sleep deprivation we feel because of British Summer Time that changes by one hour has a huge effect on our well-being. Our sleep cycle is incredibly sensitive to change and a neuroscientist at Washington University said that this adjustment corresponds with a significant increase in traffic accidents and heart attacks over the next two to three days. In the autumn when we have the extra hours of sleep, because we have put the clock back again, does not mean we are getting more sleep because overall we are sleep deprived for the few days before.

### When is the best time to sleep?

Getting to sleep before midnight has the effect of doubling the number of hours you actually sleep so that means that getting the same 8 hours of sleep from 12pm to 8am is not as beneficial as sleeping from 10pm to 6am because from 10pm to 12pm you get double the benefit as if you have slept four hours instead of two.

### What's the best temperature for sleep?

Temperatures for optimal sleep should be within 15 to 18 degrees Celsius and anything outside that range will cause difficulty in getting to sleep and staying asleep. Bathing before bed helps with sleep because the heat from the bath is lowered as soon as you get out of the bath and this is a signal to your body that it is time to go to bed.

# CHAPTER 6
# Looking After The Terrain

## Terrain is built on pH balance

To live a long and vibrant life with all your faculties and still firing on all cylinders takes a strong inner eco-system. How do we strengthen the terrain, with food and lifestyle habits? You can start from the beginning when you are in the womb. All the following principles in this chapter are built on a foundation of pH balance. What is pH? It is a scale that measures how acidic a solution is compared to how alkaline a solution is. The range is from 14, the most alkaline value, to zero, which is the most acidic value with 7 being in the middle. Humans need to have a range of somewhere in between for great health. Different parts of the human body need different levels of acidity/alkalinity to be optimally healthy for example the skin pH is 6, the stomach pH is 2 to 3, which is very acidic in order to break down protein. Blood pH is in a very narrow range of 7.35-7.45 and anything outside that range will cause you to become very ill. Blood acidity of 7.0 will kill you. Most of the metabolic processes are conducted in the blood plasma and need to be within the above ranges or they cannot happen. Let's look at an example. Oxygen cannot survive in an acidic environment so as the blood becomes more acidic oxygen will deplete. The body therefore has to make sure the acid levels of the blood stay very stable and will do anything it can to make sure that happens. Much of what we eat and drink is very acid forming and this causes inflammation. Remember, inflammation is our best defence against microbes or substances that can harm us, but too much inflammation will cause disease. That is where the saying "inflammation is the basis of all disease" comes from. You can also say "acid is the basis of all disease" because acid causes inflammation.

## Low pH and calcium

What does the body do to protect us against the acidic diet that we eat? It goes to the biggest alkaline source of minerals in the body, the calcium in the bones, and dumps calcium in the blood to put out the acid fire. There are other sources of alkaline minerals that can also be utilised but calcium in the bone is the biggest one. Having dealt with the acid fire and now everything is cooled down, the calcium will have to be dispersed throughout the body and deposited in soft tissue like the lining of the arteries causing calcification, and the acid is moved out of the blood and into the cell. It could also deposit in the kidneys causing kidney stones, the brain and breasts causing lumps.

You don't want calcium to form lumps in your breast or your brain because that would alert the powers that be to suspect cancer when it is just a benign calcium deposit. One reason why you should never take calcium supplements on their own is because it can cause these kinds of problems because you cannot direct that calcium into your bones, it can go anywhere.

## Dangers of artificial sugars

In order to keep the terrain at its best we must be careful of the amount of acidic food and drink we consume. What is acidic food? Animal products are very acidic, as well as processed foods. The most alkaline foods are the fresh plant based foods that are ideally eaten as close to their source as possible, with as little processing as possible. Fizzy drinks are one of the quickest ways to get osteoporosis. It's like drinking battery acid. We don't want any artificial sugars, they are much worse than normal sugar, especially aspartame, which causes at least 90 different chronic diseases and birth defects. It took Monsanto decades of trying to get it approved after it was rejected multiple times over fears of brain tumours and cancer. Despite aspartame killing and sickening thousands of lab animals, it was still approved to go into our drinks and chewing gum and other foods.

Michael J. Fox was a huge drinker of diet coke before he got diagnosed with Parkinson's

Aspartame is just one of the many thousands of toxins that kill us slowly, so what I am trying to say is, know exactly what you are putting in your mouth and on your skin and also know what you are breathing in as the air fresheners and perfumes we wear are full of phthalates and parabens, both made from petroleum. Diet drinks are generally loaded with Aspartame. They are harmful to humans because they disrupt our hormones and can cause allergic reactions and damage to sperm. They also accumulate in human fat tissue and over 98% of women with breast cancer have been found to have them in their breast tissue. The perfume industry is not well regulated and they don't have to disclose all the ingredients for competitive reasons.

### Dangers of using a microwave

Some things are rather obvious and using a microwave is one of them because radio frequency is used to heat food and as it does so, it changes the molecules of the food to something that the body does not recognise, an inflammatory food, and if you heat the food in a plastic container you also get some of that plastic in your food. Standing next to the microwave when it is on also exposes you to microwaves.

## The germ theory

What did Louis Pasteur say about the germ theory? He said that small bacteria that are too small to see with the naked eye are the cause of the diseases we face. Pasteur later back tracked on the germ theory when he realised it's not the bacteria, it's the terrain, otherwise why is it possible that 20 people can all get exposed to the same pathogen and only a few of them will succumb to that pathogen. The reason is that they all have immune systems that differ in strength, so if your system is strong it will not be suitable for pathogens to survive because it is healthy, then they won't thrive.

## Starting from the beginning

Looking after the terrain can start before you are born. Your parents are responsible for keeping you safe from the 80,000 different chemicals that have been produced since the 2$^{nd}$ World War. It's only since then that chemicals have been used worldwide. There is such a thing as the body burden where they are finding that on average babies are born with between 125 and 370 different toxic chemicals in their blood. Women of child bearing age should really be carefully trying to reduce their toxic burden and make sure they have an optimal level of nutrition; so that when they do happen to get pregnant they don't dump all their toxins into the baby and wonder why their baby has neurological problems or why they have had a miscarriage. When a baby has a high level of chemicals in its system it can have an immense effect on its brain and neurological development, its gut function, reducing its immune system and it makes you wonder how babies are getting cancer at such a young age.

Men also need to be healthy because their sperm affects the developing child. It takes two healthy people to produce a healthy baby.

## Feeding baby the best

Mother's milk is the best thing you can feed your baby, because it was designed that way to give your baby exactly what it needs, so making sure that your milk is of the best quality is appropriate. Formula can never compete with real breast milk, besides, most of it has got soya in it and that stops the absorption of minerals and in this day and age it's mostly GMO (Genetically Modified Organisms) as well. What else can we do to make sure our offspring start off in life with their best foot forward. Drugs and chemicals are off the menu and that includes the flu jab. The flu jab is a new development because before 2010 it was advised for pregnant women to avoid vaccinations because it was too dangerous for the developing foetus and then all of a sudden because of the H1N1 "epidemic", which is the "swine flu" where they claimed 36 pregnant women died during 2009-2012 because of the flu, they changed their mind and started vaccinating pregnant women. It's hardly justification for injecting a host of foreign substances into over 300,000 pregnant women a year in the UK alone. The reason that they were cautious about vaccinating pregnant women prior to 2010 still stands. Those jabs have over 100 different ingredients and the most damaging is mercury, which, when it is injected into the developing foetal brain, will reduce IQ, and cause other problems in the brain, because mercury is a neurotoxin (toxic to the nerves). The flu jab contains 25,000 times more mercury than the safety limit for water. The flu jab is more dangerous than the flu. They hype up the flu death numbers to scare you into getting the jab. All I know is most of the people that I spoke to about the flu jab said that they were really ill after it, including my aunty. The very concept of having to inject chemicals into you to avoid a disease that you might not get anyway, suggests that we are broken and need fixing and man knows better than nature.

## Normal birth colonization

Coming down the birth canal is the start of the baby's microbial colonisation where it is seeded with the bacteria not only from the mother but from the grandmother and great grandmother before that. This helps the baby develop a good immunity and have less allergies and autoimmune diseases. Caesarean births on the other hand only get bacteria from the microbes in the hospital environment, which is six times less bacteria than the normal birth.

So now your baby is set up with a strong set of microbes and is going to be breast fed and that will also add more beneficial microbes to baby. Breast milk is only as good as the food and toxins that you, the mother, consume so it's good to be vigilant and keep yourself healthy. The longer you breast feed the stronger the baby's immune system, up to about 3 years maximum when all the teeth should be fully present. At that age the baby is no longer producing the enzymes that can break down the protein in the milk, or the sugar in the milk and they can no longer digest Galactose in the milk. A full set of teeth means that the baby is no longer producing those enzymes so breast feeding is not an option anymore.

## Milk is species specific

All mammals produce milk that is species appropriate and perfect for their young. Goat's produce milk for their kids. Cows produce milk for their calves. Dogs produce milk for their puppies. Cows produce the milk that enables their calves to grow by 2 to 2.5 lbs per day and put on 1000-1800 lbs in two years. That is a phenomenal amount of growing and to facilitate that, cow's milk needs to have a high amount of protein, which is far beyond what humans need to be healthy. A high protein diet is stressful on your kidneys and liver because these two organs have to deal with it all.

Omega 3 is lacking in cow's milk because cows don't need to do maths and English and human babies need Omega 3 to develop their brain's properly.

How do you continue to maintain a strong terrain for your baby's health? Avoid all toxins and that means vaccines as well as chemicals and give optimal nutrition. The best way to build a strong terrain is the natural way. Your baby can taste the food you eat through the breast milk and it gets used to these tastes before birth. That is why many mothers are surprised to see that their baby seems to like the same food they like. If you want your child to eat lots of vegetables then you can eat lots of vegetables to increase the likelihood of them liking veggies.

## Listen to your biological clock

For the first few years feeding your child little and often is good because they are growing fast. By the time your little one is going to school convention says that we should be eating 3 meals a day, breakfast, dinner and tea or breakfast, lunch and dinner depending on which part of the country you live. The reason for this 3 meals a day is because when we follow the food pyramid as we are directed we will be eating a lot of cereals, grains, bread, starches, sugar with every meal. This type of food causes your sugar levels to spike very high and what goes up must come down and as it comes down you want to eat again. In order to try to stabilize the sugar levels in your blood, the advice is to eat again as soon as your sugar level starts to plummet because ideally we all need a stable sugar level all the time. We are also told to eat like a king at breakfast and eat like a pauper at night. The thing is this advice mostly ignores our biological clock, which keeps us in rhythm and in tune with everything. Our biological clock tells us when it's time to go to bed and when it's time to get up; with the sun. That is not all that is in sync with the sun, our digestive enzymes, without which we cannot break down and absorb our food is in sync with the sun. Conventional wisdom is correct when it says "don't eat late at night" because our enzymes are very low later in the evening as the sun goes down and that is why eating after 7pm means your food stays in your stomach for much longer and could still be there in the morning with some people. Midday when the sun is at its highest is when our enzymes are at their highest so that is when we should be eating our heaviest meal. In the morning our enzymes are just coming up so we need to wait but also our system is spring cleaning and performing maintenance on all the cells, especially our brain from 4am – 12pm and when you start to eat you stop this process. If you are used to skipping breakfast don't be concerned, as long as you are not eating too late in the night you should be ok.

Everything we were taught from school and in conventional circles is generally the opposite of what is true. If they tell us one thing, turn it upside down and you will be closer to the truth.

## Avoiding chemicals

This is not easy because they are pervasive and ubiquitous and half the time you don't even realise there is a harmful chemical in a product because it's a cleaning fluid that you have used all your life. What exactly is a chemical? Generally a chemical is a substance that is not found in nature so it has been made in a lab. Take the everyday bleaches and disinfectants and baby lotions and talcum powders, detergents, plastic bottles. We have been using these products for so long without question because we believe what the adverts tell us, but they are not telling us the other side of the coin, what harm these products can also cause.

The body does not know what to do with chemicals. Chemicals block your pathways and destroy your enzymes so they are always harmful and they always cause side effects, even Aspirin, and man has created a toxic world. Toxins are in the air we breathe, the water we drink, the food we eat and it is impossible to get away from all of them. All we can do is reduce our toxic burden as much as possible. There is a lot we can do so don't give up.

## Non-food, food

Here in the west we have a tendency to be malnourished and overweight at the same time. Your body is demanding more food because the "food" that it has received so far has not been satisfying or nutritious and it is in fact starving you of good quality nutrition and will make you eat and eat in the hope that you will give it something it can use. Heating and processing the food tends to kill the atoms and molecules that are in the food and they cannot help the body thrive at all instead they cause disease and sickness.

## Unclog the organs

How do we get a strong immune system, by lightening the load on your organs and you do that by cleaning them out. If your organs are clogged up with heavy metals or silted up with salt or mucus causing foods they will struggle to perform. It will be like wading through treacle for them. Efficient organs are clean organs. Yes you can clean out your insides just the same as you can clean your outsides and it is something we should do regularly at the very least once a year but ideally 4 times a year if we want to remain strong.

## Alternative to antibiotics

Antibiotics are chemicals that indiscriminately kill off all the bacteria, especially your gut bacteria that you need, so why do it to yourself, when there are alternatives. An unknown side effect of taking antibiotics is getting thrush soon afterwards. Ask your doctor or nurse why you get thrush and they will tell you because the gut bacteria has been put out of balance. Instead of using antibiotics, garlic has been known to do a wonderful job of neutralizing harmful bacteria. It has 34 natural antibiotics with no known side effects except for it being a little hot for some people. Colloidal silver is another alternative to antibiotics. Food grade hydrogen peroxide is another supplement you can use, just stick to the stated dose and don't overdo it. Organic essential oils are anti-viral, anti-fungal, and anti-bacterial. Some are stronger than others and Oregano is very strong and effective and also Frankincense. Dependence on antibiotics is not necessary especially when the alternatives work much better.

## Why we don't want Wi-Fi

Protect your house against radio waves and electromagnetic energy. Sensitive people get very ill with Smart Meters, which are not smart at all. They call them Smart Meters so that people will get them installed just to prove how smart they are. Question everything, especially why they are giving things away for free. These meters can make you so sick that you become disabled and have to stop work. If you have a smart meter you need to know that they continually emit radiation every few seconds so the signals pass straight through your walls and your own body and other objects. Smart meters will synchronize together and become more powerful than the individual meters. For example, if there are three meters on your street, the strength of those three meters will form a much stronger network and it will be as if there are five meters. There is no legal requirement to have a smart meter for an individual residential property or for a business property. Symptoms such as migraines, insomnia, memory loss, fatigue, heart palpitations, loss of balance and many more neurological problems have been reported as well as increasing your risk of developing cancer.

## Toxic air in your home

Your home may be your castle but with the off gassing of all the chemicals into your atmosphere at home, it is far more toxic than the air outside. Fire retardants outgas from your furniture, mattresses, carpets, blinds, children's nightclothes, electronics casing, electric wires and cables, and building insulation. These chemical effects on health far out-weigh any perceived benefits and can cause disrupted hormones, reduced fertility, interference in the developing brain, neurological defects and have been found in human blood, fat and breast milk around the world. Dust on the floor where children play also contains flame retardants and children tend to have higher concentrations of flame retardants in their body than adults. Cooking with non-stick pans also adds toxins to the air in your home. They cause health effects over many years rather than immediately.

## If you can't eat it, forget it

The most used chemicals are the ones that we think are harmless. We have all sorts of cleaning fluids for every surface, cleaners for glass surfaces, for the bath, for wooden floors for steel surfaces, for furniture. The more surfaces there are the more cleaning fluids we have. The truth is you can use one cleaner for all of them and that cleaner would be very natural and something that we can actually consume without any harm. We need a cleaner that, when we wash it down the sink into the sewer, it is totally harmless to the environment and to the ecosystem. Pesticides used on weeds, not only pollute the air and the soil and the water but will poison everything in the ecosystem and is not needed because there are always safe and effective alternatives. As we poison the sea the fish become poisoned and we eat the fish so it is a vicious cycle.

## Clean up your bedroom

Considering that we spend eight or so hours a day in our bed, which is one third of our life, it stands to reason that it is important to get a comfortable bed and it is even more important to make sure that the bed is safe to sleep on. A memory foam mattress off gasses a dense chemical substance, which only adds to the chemical soup that we live in day to day. Not only the mattress but the pillow can also be made of toxic chemicals and the sheets are normally made of synthetic substances that off gas if it is not made from organic material. It is perfectly legal for the bedding companies to poison us with impunity. This also applies to our clothing. Samina organic beds are better.

## Our clothes can kill us

The clothing we wear today, along with the dyes, has documented threats to our health and environment. Clothing made from synthetic fibre hides invisible chemicals that most of the health care industry ignores. Natural fibres were the norm until the petrochemical revolution in the early 20th century when synthetic fibres were invented; the first one being Nylon made out of petroleum by Dupont, a chemist. He was the father of the synthetic textile industry. Today we have "wash and wear" fabrics made from acrylic, the "wrinkle free" fabrics made from xylene and ethylene. Spandex for stretchiness created for sport and swimming. The dyes are also derived from petroleum and the industry is well known for decimating and destroying vast ecosystems. Nowadays there are about 8000 chemicals used on each item of clothing from start to finish that includes the cleaning, bleaching, washing, dry cleaning, dying, scouring, finishing. The chemicals include things like formaldehyde, flame retardants and chemicals to make them wrinkle free. They add nano-particles to clothes and they are so tiny that they get into the DNA of humans, animals and plant life causing dangerous effects.

One of the most toxic textiles today is cotton because it is saturated with pesticides and fertilizers (1/3lb per tee shirt) and most of them are GMO's (genetically modified organisms) because they will off gas and those GMO's are linked to autism, Parkinson's, cancer and hormone disruption. Many of the GMO cotton is responsible for over 300,000 Indian farmer suicides because the promise that GMO's would make them rich by giving a huge yield had quite the opposite effect and they drank the Round-up because it was the only way that they could see to get out of the debt that these crops caused.

# CHAPTER 7
# Vitamin D

## Importance of Vitamin D

Vitamin D is essential for maintaining our health and it will not be produced by the body without adequate amounts of essential omega 3 fatty acids. Your body has receptors on every cell for vitamin D, which means it must be pretty important.

## Vitamin D is a hormone

Hormone D would be more accurate because it is a hormone. Why is it a hormone? Because it is a chemical messenger that occurs naturally in our body, and travels through the blood, to certain cells to tell them what to do. Why is Hormone D so important? Without it nothing else will work properly. Hormone D is involved in every process that goes on in the body. It is synthesized by sunlight on the skin. Hormone D courses through our blood and helps with the following:-

- Helps to repair all our organs
- Increases muscle tone
- Regulates and boosts hormones
- Organises our bio-chemical processes
- Relaxes our nerves
- Supports our eye health
- Increases oxygen levels of the blood and tissue
- Regulates basal metabolic rate
- Repairs DNA
- Is good for your thyroid
- Boosts your immune system
- Maintains healthy skin
- Helps kill bacteria
- Produces cholesterol sulphate
- Lowers blood sugar
- Lowers blood pressure
- Hormone D protects against sun burn
- Helps to strengthen bones

So you can see how serious and absolutely essential hormone D is. It should be the first consideration of all health care professionals, because low levels of hormone D are linked to, depression, asthma, cancer, osteoporosis, dementia, autism, muscular sclerosis, diabetes, high blood pressure, psoriasis and a host more. Many people get the idea that the sun causes skin cancer so they slap on the sun screen. When the sun burns those sun screen chemicals into your skin it is far worse off than just getting sunburn because your body can cope with that, but those chemicals that have no place in a human may stay lodged in your fat for years, if you are lucky. If not you could get ill.

There are two different types of UV rays. UVB rays are the beneficial ones that give you hormone D and they also protect against melanoma, the worst kind of skin cancer. UVA rays are not responsible for your hormone D or your tanned skin. It is the UVA rays that cause cancer and the sun screens typically block the UVB good rays and let the UVA dangerous rays in to cause havoc.

### How do we get hormone D?

The best way to get it is by getting the sun on your skin. Mushrooms apparently contain it so you can eat them but you won't get enough. Safe tanning beds are another way to get it and you can also supplement. Not everyone on the planet is exposed to a lot of sunshine. If you are lucky enough to live within 5000 miles of the equator, your sun exposure will be significant. When the sky is cloudy, the sun rays find it harder to get through so the energy intensity will be lower. Skin exposure matters, the more skin exposed the more hormone D you produce.

How much hormone D do we need every day? Doctors tell us that 2000 IU is the maximum we should take. They are not considering your optimal health, they are considering the minimum necessary to prevent rickets. 30 minutes of natural sun exposure can increase hormone D by up to 35,000 IU. Other consultants say 10,000 IU will get you up to the right level if you are short and 5,000 IU will keep you stable.

# CHAPTER 8
# Exercise

### Exercise, can you be healthy without it?

What benefits do we give our body by exercising? Movement of our muscles increases heat and causes sweating thereby allowing the toxins to be excreted through the skin. The lymph system is the bodies sewage system and it has four times more lymph vessels than blood vessels (what is that telling you?) but they don't have a pump and the only way we can move the lymph around is by moving our muscles or jumping on a trampoline where gravity squeezes these lymph vessels and speeds up the elimination of the toxins through the blood. Lack of movement means that the lymph vessels accumulate toxins and keep them in the body depressing our immune system.

## Exercise benefits the muscles

Exercise strengthens the muscles, ligaments and tendons around our joints helping them to stay strong and supported and reducing pain, as long as we are not overdoing it, causing them to tear. High blood pressure can be reduced by exercise because as you increase your exercise you are increasing the demand on the heart and the blood vessels have to dilate in order for more blood to travel to where it is needed and your body gets used to this increase in demand over time. Walking up stairs will demand more energy and oxygen than when you are walking on a flat surface so the more you do this the easier it will be for your blood vessels to adapt. Insomnia can be improved by exercising because it makes you more tired so you can sleep better at night. Heavy exercise such as HIIT (High Intensity Interval Training) or weights will brings out the Human Growth Hormone (HGH) that causes more activity in the cells because they are repairing and that will also tire you out and make it easier to sleep so playing hard helps you to sleep hard. Strong muscles and joints will improve your posture making your overall look healthier and appealing, not to mention keeping you energized and ready to go. Starting exercise early on in life will more than likely mean you carry on into adulthood and bones will adapt to stress and become stronger so if you are exercising from a young age you are continually strengthening your bones and warding off osteoporosis.

## Exercise is good for the joints

Joint lubrication is induced by the synovial membrane that produces synovial fluid that washes over the joint when it is moved and it is like oiling an engine that stops your bones grinding on one another. The joint gets nourished, oxygenated and lubricated. To fully lubricate the joint you need to take that joint through its full range of motion. If you are continually extending your elbow by 80% then there will be 20% of the joint that does not get nourished and metabolites will build up causing arthritis or debris to build up in the joint. What do they say about your body? If you don't use it you lose it and that is exactly what will happen. Many body builders who use heavy weights are prone to not fully extending their elbows because they are scared that the weight will be too heavy and turn their elbow inside out. They never fully extend the elbow joint and pretty soon the bicep muscle shortens and then they find that they can't extend it and the elbow remains permanently bent. Over a period of time the elbow joint will get painful and arthritic. Not all joints are synovial joints but all joints need to move through their full range of motion in order to keep them flexible.

## Exercise is good for the nerves

Our bodies are not designed to be sedentary at all. Sitting for a few minutes is okay but nowadays we are sitting more than we are standing. Our heart pumps our blood around but we also need to move around for the blood to circulate properly. The nerves also benefit from movement. Why? Because they get more blood supply when we move and they are activating metabolic processes. More blood creates new nerve growth, increased nerve interconnections and maintenance of the nerves. Every cell gets more blood supply when we move even those areas that do not have their own blood supply like the joint cartilages. They get their blood supply from the surrounding tissue so it is more important for them to move.

## Sitting is the new smoking

Blood and the blood vessels are the transport system that deliver oxygen and nutrition to every cell and take out the trash, making all cells more robust. Sitting will slow everything down and the electrical energy of the muscles also slows right down as soon as we sit causing muscles to atrophy over time, meaning to waste away. Even if you exercise every day as soon as you sit the deterioration begins again in proportion to the amount of time you sit. Sitting also decreases insulin sensitivity, which means your cells are not sensitive to insulin anymore and you need far more insulin to get the job done (put glucose into the cell for energy) increasing your risk of developing Type II diabetes.

How you sit has a role in the quality of your health. Sitting is the new smoking. Most of the modern day chairs force the spine into a poor position, especially in the lumbar area, causing a slouching with shoulders rolled forward and the spine shaped like a letter C instead of its natural S shape putting extra pressure on the spinal discs and the spinal bones, causing adaptation in those bones that changes their shape, leading to more problems. The spinal bones are there to support our structure and protect the central nerves which travel along them so if they are not shaped correctly blockages can easily happen. Sciatica being a good example of how this can happen. Sciatica is one of the most common back problems many people suffer from, where they get back pain that travels all the way down the back of the legs. The sciatic nerve, being the thickest nerve in the body, is the easiest to get compressed because of its size and its position being at the bottom of the spine so all the weight of gravity from the top of the spine can effect it.

A spine shaped like the letter C puts compression through your lungs as you bend forward so that you can't breathe properly because you can't fill them up with air.

Our muscles are all covered by a fine layer of fascia. Fascia is a tough sheet of connective tissue that is as strong as tensile steel. It is below the skin and it surrounds the muscles and organs to secure them into place and to keep them separated from each other. Fascia can reform itself and it loves to be masterfully lead but if you neglect it by sitting a lot, it will grow thicker and stiffer. When we sit for long periods of time, such as 20 minutes or more, the fascia that surrounds the muscle adapts to the shape that it is in and it wrecks your hip action by tightening the hip flexors, the muscles at the front of the hip. Tight hip flexors makes it more difficult to swing your leg backwards so you have a shorter step and a reduced balance. Elders have got a characteristic posture that is caused by the accumulation of decades of sitting. If you want to maintain your flexibility long term sitting is not advised. A sedentary lifestyle is a health risk that is as high as smoking and obesity because we were not designed to be sedentary at all.

The easier you find it to sit down on the floor and get back up again without having to use your hands, the longer you are predicted to live. So if you are stiff, don't worry, you can do something about it. Gently stretch your muscles and hold the stretch for at least 30 seconds and that will stretch the fascia. Keeping your legs working as in standing for long periods of time is beneficial because it keeps your heart working and your muscles engaged. Standing still is only so effective because movement is the key. Changing your posture continually throughout the day as in standing on one leg then the other is what you need. When sitting keep your pelvic bowl tilted forward so that your low back has an S shape. Standing desks are becoming more and more popular as people begin to realise the benefits of standing without there being an adverse impact on production.

Sitting for too long, too often, has an effect of shortening your overall lifespan. Have you ever seen a 4 year old who has back pain from too much sitting? Maybe we should be getting back the movement we once had as children, when we would squat right down when we are focused on doing something like making a sand castle, rather than sitting in a chair. We should be able to move without fear of injury and use our body to its full potential. If we move in the way our body is designed to move then toned muscles and a slimmer physique would be inevitable. Sitting for 10 hours a day sets you back so much that even if you work out for an hour afterwards it will not fully reverse the effects.

Many times when we want to look good we focus on the muscles and start doing weights instead of focusing on the movement and the movement recruits the muscles. The Chinese believe you are only as old as your spine. Sitting creates stasis as blood pools in the body. Perhaps if you focus on moving the spine by gently bending the spine every day through four different planes it would benefit your health. Backwards forward, up and down, side bends and side twists.

## Is sleeping bad too?

What about when you are sleeping? We are designed to rest and recuperate so when we are laying down and sleeping our metabolic processes are very low and our heart is not stressed so that we are not effected in the same way as when we sit in the daytime.

## Exercise and the micro biome

Exercise can improve the micro biome on its own without changing anything else. You can't exercise your way out of a bad diet but it can increase good bacteria that reduces inflammation and help prevent cancer and also boosts your metabolism.

## Exercise slows ageing

Exercise can hold back some of the negative impacts of ageing like memory loss. Sarcopenia in the older adult (40 plus), which is muscle atrophy, is not inevitable and can be stopped by regular exercise, such as weights, as well as aerobics. Planned exercise can help but so can some aspects of daily living such as walking instead of taking the bus. Aerobic fitness or maximum oxygen consumption will naturally decrease as we age but not so much if we continue to exercise and aerobic exercise is a kind of exercise that anybody at any age can start. 80 year olds who have not been used to regular exercise, actually start training for marathons and run the whole 26 miles. Older people who exercise can have a profile the same as people who are in their 20's and 30's. There is evidence that exercise can also decrease your risk of getting a degenerative disease such as diabetes, high blood pressure, arthritis, cardiovascular disease and cancer. Blood sugar is maintained better when people exercise and eat well. Exercise reduces the amount of triglycerides in their blood, which is fat in the blood, and it reduces their likelihood of having a heart attack or stroke because the blood is not as thick. As people get older they generally do less exercise and then they blame their ailments on getting older, when it is actually caused by lack of exercise and improper nutrition because age is not a disease. If they start to exercise and eat well they could reduce their medication and that means less side effects, making them feel better, then they might be more enthusiastic about exercising and it is a vicious cycle. Even if you are on many medications and have plenty of chronic illnesses you can still improve with exercise.

### Exercise helps dementia

Dementia, the most common of which is Alzheimer's, benefits greatly by movement especially aerobic movement because blood and oxygen are both pumped to the brain as well as other nutrients that is in the blood keeping your brain more alert. Aerobic exercise benefits many psychiatric disorders and is much underused as a treatment. It can help with depression, anxiety, and chronic pain because of endorphins, which is the high you get when you exercise and endorphins reduce your stress hormones. It improves learning and memory and it improves your ability to differentiate between different faces.

Increasing your steps to at least 10,000 a day from the average 3,500 a day will really improve your health.

## How to reduce your sitting time

First find out how long you are sitting every day, then take steps to reduce it. How do you make exercise a convenient part of your life? By planning ahead, making it fun and enjoyable and slotting it into your lifestyle. It must be easy to access, like standing up for five minutes every half hour while you are at work, doing some simple exercises at your desk, getting off the bus two stops earlier than usual, taking the stairs at work, parking your car two blocks away or making a commitment to always get up and pace up and down when you are on the phone. Performing exercises that are efficient and tend to use more muscle groups in your body, such as a bicep curl with squats, then why would you just do the squats on their own when you can engage all the muscles of the body instead of just the lower half. Use enough effort in your exercises so that you can feel a difference. Even if you just fidget, that can be a benefit by reducing your mortality. Monitor your progress and make sure you record it because if you are not seeing any results you won't keep it up. Once you get into the habit it will become second nature.

## Breathing for vitality

Breathing exercises can also be a benefit for cardiovascular health as they open up the muscles in between the ribs causing proper oxygenation, relaxation and focus. Without even noticing, most of us do not breathe properly and only use half the capacity of our lungs. Five minutes a day of deep conscious breathing can make all the difference to your day and your life.

# CHAPTER 9
# Fasting

## What is fasting?

Fasting literally means to not eat for an extended period of time. So you are deliberately depriving yourself of food in order to get the benefits that you want to get. There are many different reasons that people fast and all religions have a period of fasting as a concept of being closer to spirit. Christians have Lent, Muslims have Ramadan, and Jews have Shabbat and so on. There are other reasons for fasting apart from spiritual enlightenment.

Fasting benefits are:-

- Rest from working on digestion
- Increase lifespan
- Can get you into a ketogenic state to improve health

- Fasting and weight loss
- Fasting cures diseases
- Diabetes
- Alzheimers
- Epilepsy
- Cancer
- Eyesight

Give the body a rest from digestion. It is a very hard working process for the body. Digestion consumes about 60% of the bodies overall energy and many times we start eating early in the morning until late at night making it work for about 16 hours none stop without realising the heavy toll we are placing on our body's resources. If the body is using less energy by breaking down less food then that means it can get on with other jobs it has to do like cleaning house and looking after the immune system.

Fasting or calorie restriction is the number one best way to add years to your life. There is no food you can eat, no drink you can drink, no exercise you can have, or any pill you can take; there is nothing else you can do that extends your life more than calorie restriction. There have been experiments on mice, rats, monkeys, yeast, flies and worms and they have found the same thing. Reduce calories by 20% and they all live longer.

## Why would anyone want to get into ketosis?

Ketosis is when your body burns fat instead of carbohydrates and your liver makes ketone bodies, Your body can burn carbohydrates (definition of carbohydrates is sugar both natural and unnatural, including fruit and starchy vegetables, starches like bread, pasta, potatoes, rice and grains are also carbohydrates because they turn to sugar very quickly before they hit the stomach) for fuel or fat for fuel. When you keep your carbohydrates low and the body is in starvation mode the body switches to burning the fat instead. Your liver converts that fat into energy molecules called ketone bodies. Ketones are able to increase athletic performance by about 2%, which makes all the difference to an Olympic athlete. You can be a sugar burner and still burn a little bit of fat. You can be a fat burner and still burn a little bit of sugar. What determines which one you are, is insulin. When insulin enters the cell it blocks fat from being used, then all you have got is sugar so you are a sugar burner. Sugar produces a lot of by-products, a lot of smoke, a lot of ash, a lot of embers. It burns very hot and produces a lot of free radicals. It triggers hormones, cortisol, thyroid, and insulin and oestrogen hormones. These hormones when in the presence of free radicals caused by sugar burning will lead to accelerated ageing, disease and pain. The sugar causes extra soot, extra ash and your cells don't repair as well. Oxidation and reduced energy can cause chronic fatigue, brain fog and metabolic down regulation. In combination with the hormones the oxidative stress leads to inflammation. Inflammation is joint pain, muscle pain, auto-immune issues and all sorts of chronic diseases. If you get rid of the insulin that will open up the fat burning pathway. Fat burning is like a nice clean blue flame, that burns consistently and steadily with no by products, very little smell, no smoke and is very efficient so suddenly now your cell can upgrade its function and be robust with good protection and repair and you have loads of energy. Hydroxybuterate, which is created during fat burning, is the most efficient fuel source known to man. Free radicals are 50 times less as a fat burner than when you are burning sugar. The hormones produced during fat burning are Human Growth Hormone (fountain of youth), DHEA, (DHEA is a massive anti-stress, repair and longevity hormone) testosterone (for increased muscle mass, lean body, strong bones and boosted sex drive), adrenaline for good mental clarity and get out of bed hormone and oxytocin, the loving, connection, friendship, relationship hormone that kills all the negative hormones cortisol, oestrogen, insulin and thyroid. Cortisol is the killer stress hormone and oxytocin is its natural antidote. Sugar burning promotes disease, stress, ageing and pain. Fat burning promotes youth, longevity, health, mental clarity and high energy.

## Carbohydrates and gaining weight

Fasting means eating less food so restricting the amount you eat will help with weight loss especially if you are restricting carbohydrates. Carbohydrates are the main culprit for putting on weight.

## Benefits of calorie restriction

Calorie restriction decreases blood pressure, triglycerides, atherosclerotic plaque, insulin resistance and increases insulin sensitivity. Calorie restriction will decrease glucose levels in the blood because if the insulin resistance is reduced then more of the glucose can travel from the blood into the cell and the pancreas does not have to make as much insulin, reducing its work load. Calorie restriction also reduces the proliferation of cancer cells because they need energy to grow so reducing the amount of energy the cancer uses as food, reduces its progression. Cancer cells have damaged mitochondria and cannot use fat as fuel. With over 1000 metabolic processes happening in the body at any one time, the calorie restriction or fasting promotes the clearance of fat in all tissues. Fat is everywhere throughout the body and we need fat but sometimes it is getting in the way of healthy processes like for example too much unhealthy fat around each cell is what causes insulin resistance and when we reduce that, the insulin can work better by getting sugar in the cell and diabetes is improved or eliminated altogether. Calorie restriction will benefit people with kidney problems, multiple sclerosis, heart disease, autism and will help body builders build more muscle and other benefits.

## The many different ways of fasting

Water fast is where you consume water and nothing else for the duration of the fast. Water fasts are easier to do than a completely dry fast and can be continued for a longer period of time because the body can continue for a few weeks without food, and water will sustain you for a short while because the cells are still getting what they want to be able to perform the many metabolic processes that they need to do and they can normally use the reserves of fat and nutrition that are already in the body.

Dry fast is the harshest of all fasts where you let nothing at all pass through your lips and should not be undertaken lightly or for long periods of time. I think the body can survive about 10 days without water so you would not dry fast for that long. Five days is the maximum to be going without water but your kidneys get slightly damaged when you are dehydrated because they are working hard to balance the blood pressure and the solutes in the blood.

Intermittent fasting. There are various ways to do this. You can fast for one day on and one day off or for five days a week then eat at the weekends or vice versa and eat for five days a week then fast at the weekends. You can fast on a daily basis where you restrict your eating window to eight hours a day by fasting up till 11am or 12pm then you start eating up till 7pm or 8pm when you stop eating and that incurs 16 hours of not eating until the next day or you can just have one meal a day and fast for 22 to 23 hours every day. When you don't eat for long periods of time it can take you into ketosis and that is where most of the health benefits lie. You can fast for five days out of every month and still get some benefit.

## Benefits of a detox

The best minerals for the human to consume are those that you get from vegetables, fruits, nuts, seeds and herbs. Unfortunately, in this day and age, we are consuming, breathing in and absorbing through our skin huge amounts of toxins and chemicals that harm us both short and long term. Even when we are eating the right food we have commissioned outsiders to grow our food and have to trust that they are growing it in a healthy way. Our liver and organs are equipped to clean out our system but with the barrage of chemicals that have entered our lives in the last 60 years our liver is struggling to keep our head above water. The body gets rid of toxins through our skin, intestines, kidneys and lymph system so we want to make sure that these systems of elimination are clear. Detoxification helps to strengthen the immune system and fights off infection. Toxins are stored in your fat cells so when you want to lose weight it can be very difficult because the body does not want to dump those toxins from the fat into the blood potentially causing disease or illness. When you clean your organs you can get rid of many issues of bloating, nausea, mood swings, boost energy, reduce pain and many symptoms and it creates a more efficient detox.

How often do you need to detox because if you detoxify for too long you can lose valuable nutrients along with the toxins and deplete your body. Ideally we would fast at least once a year and even better would be three times a year

If you promote the burning of fat from most of your tissues you will lose weight. If you promote the burning of fat from your liver and muscles you will increase insulin sensitivity and that helps heal diabetes and Alzheimer's because Alzheimer's is said to be diabetes Type III. If you promote the clearance of fat from your blood vessels and your heart you will reduce your risk of atherosclerosis and cardiovascular disease. A ketogenic diet along with intermittent fasting is also beneficial for epilepsy because it promotes the burning of fat from your brain cells (amyloid plaque) and then you can replace that with good fat. Cancer feeds on sugar or carbohydrates so if your diet is low in these foods, the cancer will starve, so you can also use intermittent fasting to deter cancer. The ketogenic diet is not suitable for all types of cancer.

Your eyes are very sensitive to sugar like the canary in the coal mine. Your eyesight can degenerate very quickly and fluctuate up and down moment to moment. The best thing you can do for your eyesight is to reduce the sugar, so that is where intermittent fasting or ketogenic diet will really benefit your eyes.

# CHAPTER 10
# Putting it all together

## Giving the body what it needs

This book is not just about reducing symptoms but it is also about prevention of those unnecessary chronic diseases. First of all, let's start with the fact that most of the chronic diseases we experience today are built on inflammation and getting rid of the inflammation is half the battle. With that in mind, most diseases can be prevented, can be reversed, and even cured. You just have to find the cause of the inflammation and a few other things and that will be it. Our body is a miraculous, self-healing machine, you just need to give it what it needs and it will do all the healing. Most people want to know how to be healthy and how to have great health into the distant future and it is very possible. Information is the key. Observe and copy nature as much as you can because we are natural beings so keep everything as unprocessed as possible. If you are confused about what constitutes natural then ask yourself what would happen in nature. I always go to nature for the answers.

## The importance of hydration

Understanding the importance of water will drive you to drink more of it. First thing in the morning, as soon as you get up, because you will be dehydrated after a long nights sleep, before you have your morning coffee or tea, drink the best liquid for you. Coffee and tea will dehydrate you even more. During the night there are many biological processes happening and the by-product of that is mostly acid so we want to alkalize in the morning. The best alkalizing drink is green juice and drinking green juice in the morning is like taking a big jug of supplements to set you up for the day. You are literally juicing for life because that is what it gives you, life in your cells and is well known as a way of getting rid of inflammation, used by many with chronic illnesses. Coconut water is also a good way to alkalize and hydrate. If you are drinking water for hydration then add juice from a real lemon. It sounds contradictory to add lemon juice but lemons are unique in the plant world because they are acidic when you drink the juice, but because they are so full of alkalizing minerals like calcium, potassium, and magnesium, after you have digested the lemon it will increase your alkalinity. Do not put the lemon juice in boiling water because it will kill the vitamin C. The temperature of the water needs to be warm because the body has to change the temperature to be able to use it efficiently. When the water is cold it shocks the body, especially the liver so don't give the body too much hard work to do. Just be careful when drinking the lemon juice to use a straw because it will corrode your teeth.

So what is the best water you should be drinking? Certainly not tap water. Filter your water with something stronger than a Brita Filter. Tap liquid will cause free radicals to build up in your body, causing wrinkles, ageing and disease.

## Strengthen the terrain

The body's terrain can determine how healthy or ill you become. To strengthen the terrain we want to increase the number of different bacteria we have in our gut micro biome and we do that by eating probiotics every day with our meals. These probiotics need feeding so prebiotics will fulfil that roll. What are prebiotics? They are foods that contain fibre; vegetables, fruit, nuts and seeds.

## Watch those toxic dental procedures

We want to keep a clean mouth and that also means not having any root canals because all root canals are infected and weaken our immune system. There is no way that the thousands and thousands of little tubules that run perpendicular to the main canal can be cleaned and they can destroy your enzymes when they are toxic.

## Hormone D protects your health

Hormone D builds a strong body terrain that protects against cancer. Hormone D will not be produced in the body without adequate amounts of essential omega 3 fatty acids. To protect yourself against sun burn, the more anti-oxidants you have in your system the less you burn. Hormone D must be taken with vitamin K2 because as hormone D helps calcium to absorb into the body, vitamin K2 will put the calcium where it belongs in the bones to avoid calcification elsewhere. Hormone D is a good inflammation suppressor. Have you not noticed how good you feel when you are on holiday somewhere hot and as soon as you land back home with the grey skies and grey weather you immediately feel down? Next time you are not feeling your best, consider your hormone D levels as the first port of call.

## Getting a great night sleep

Sleep is as essential as good food and is impossible to achieve without magnesium. Magnesium is involved in more than 300 different bodily processes as well as sleep and proper digestion. What is the best natural source of magnesium, green leafy vegetables like spinach, kale, water cress, parsley? There is a rising tide of insomnia as more and more people are joining this epidemic of extreme magnesium shortage. Doctors who check for magnesium will check the blood and magnesium is always balanced in the blood because otherwise death results and consequently doctors seem to think that everybody's levels of magnesium are just right, when a more thorough test would be to test the red blood cell to give a better idea. You have to demand this red blood cell test because they do not give it as a general rule. How else do we make sure we get a deep sleep? Electrical objects must be kept out of the bedroom because it should be a sleeping sanctuary. Keep the bedroom pitch black and not too hot or too cold. Install software f.lux on your pc or laptop so that you don't get blue light at night causing your circadian rhythm to be disrupted.

### Get the right equipment

Let's start with getting your home ready for healing so that means having the right equipment to make it easy for you to prepare those meals that are as close to nature as possible. We need to be eating a large portion of our food raw because when has heat ever enhanced your food? Heat destroys the enzymes that you need to digest food, which puts a lot of pressure on your pancreas in its effort to make more enzymes. When you eat a raw piece of fruit or a raw vegetable, all the enzymes that are needed to break that food down will already be in that food. It's like a ready packed meal, loaded with everything you need.

Things you need in your kitchen are blenders, juicers

and food processors and they need to be on the kitchen counter top for easy access because if they are in the cupboard you are not going to be dragging them out of the cupboard every time you want to use them. You need glass containers instead of plastic, wooden chopping boards instead of plastic because remember plastic is made from petrochemicals and is an endocrine disruptor. You also need a range of sharp knives that will cut efficiently. Make sure any pots and pans are not Teflon because although Teflon is okay when it's cold, as soon as you heat the pan up the chemicals get cooked into your food. The best pans to use are glass and ceramic or enamel. Even stainless steel pans will put small amounts of chromium and nickel in your food. Titanium pots are very expensive and still off gas toxic components into your food according to Blanche Grube, a biological dentist who warns you against putting titanium in to your root canals.

## Bye bye to processed food

Reduce the consumption of processed food and sugar and eat food that is ideally prepared at home from fresh. If you want to be full of energy you have to eat food that is full of energy. Processed food is bad for us because in order to extend the shelf life they use extreme heat which destroys a lot of the nutrition and, also, they put all kinds of unsavoury chemicals in there so that you are left with only a remnant of the real food.

## Processed food and low fertility

As each population adopts more processed food the health goes down and fertility suffers. We are all designed to have perfectly straight teeth and not get cavities. When you are eating real, nutrient-dense foods, you get the complete and perfect expression of the genetic potential. We were given a perfect blueprint. Whether or not the body is built according to the blueprint depends, to a great extent, on our wisdom in food choices. This is the terrible price of the West, the Western price. Civilization will die out unless we embrace the food that we are designed to eat. That means turning our backs on processed foods and getting back into the kitchen, to prepare real foods--containing healthy fats--for ourselves and our families. In the last 40 years human fertility has been reduced by 58%. When that figure gets to 72% they start worrying about the survival of the species.

## No irradiation thank you

Avoid food that is radiated because that also destroys between 5 and 80% of the nutrient content. Examples of radiated foods are herbs and spices, fruit and vegetables, root vegetables, cereals, poultry, fish and shellfish unless it says it's organic because you can't have any radiated, organic food. Apples that don't turn brown when they have been cut means they are radiated or they could also be GMO because there is a new GMO apple called the Arctic Apple that does not go brown when you cut it open. Vegetables that are cut up into pieces and prepacked into plastic bags are treated with chlorine to stop them from going brown. Chlorine is one of the chemicals that will devastate your ability to break down your food properly. All this attention to what we eat, drink and put in our house is all to reduce the acid levels in our blood and our cells. As humans, we want to keep our blood acid levels between 7.35 and 7.45. Anything outside that range will cause inflammation and disease. If you really want to know how your lifestyle is affecting your pH levels, get some pH sticks and measure your levels 30 minutes after eating food and you will find out how the different foods you eat affect you as an individual.

We are seeing an epidemic of allergies, auto immune diseases and chronic illness today more than ever. The more raw and fresh whole foods that you eat the more ability to detoxify and strengthen the immune system and therefore destroy harmful pathogens.

### Toxic air in your house

Opening windows or using air filters or plants that filter out toxic air is a good idea. Mopping the floor frequently or vacuuming to reduce dust is also a good idea. When buying new products buy those products that are flame retardant free and don't buy polystyrene or polyurethane

All plants absorb some of the particles in the air when they take in carbon dioxide and through photosynthesis along with microbes in the soil, break down these particles as they create the oxygen, but some plants can do that more efficiently than others. Here is a list of plants that are slightly better at detoxifying the air.

- Peace Lilly
- English Ivy
- Parlour Ivy
- African Violet
- Devil's Ivy
- Christmas Cactus
- Spider Plant
- Boston Fern
- Mother-in-Law's Tongue
- Bamboo Palm
- Aloe Vera

## Swop out the chemicals

Toxic chemicals in our home, endocrine disruptors' plastic, phthalates, PCB's are silent killers that we think are safe. Swop out your chemical cleaners for natural ones like white spirit vinegar, bicarbonate of soda, lemon juice, castile soap, food grade hydrogen peroxide or even low pH water from an ionizer. Swop out your toiletries for natural ones. If you can't eat it you should not be putting it on your skin, the biggest organ of the human body. We are paying for our own demise especially where perfumes are concerned because they generally have over 100 different chemicals in each perfume.

## Swop out your Wi-Fi

Get an Ethernet cable. Get rid of all the telephone base stations in your house because the energy is strong and damaging to your cells. Do not get a smart meter installed, even if it's free; especially if it's free. Question why they are giving these meters for free when the powers that be don't like to give anything away.

## Toxic clothes

If you are going to wear anything made from cotton or have cotton towels or mats make sure it is organic because GMO cotton is still full of glyphosate that is always off gassing even if you keep washing it. Natural fabric is the only fabric that we should be putting next to our skin, so all the rayon's, nylon's and wrinkle free fabrics are not good for us because they are continually off gassing and they don't allow our skin to breath.

## Exercise

We need to exercise on a daily basis even if it's only walking. Choose the exercise that you will regularly do, something that you enjoy, that way it is not a chore. If you can't do some form of exercise daily then do a minimum of three times a week as long as it's regular and part of your lifestyle.

## Detoxify or die

After all the physical toxins and emotional toxins that can build up and wreck our health we need to detoxify at least once a year and reset our system and start again. Colon cleanse is the first place to start because we have to clean out the pathway of illumination for everything to come out. Next is the liver because the two together builds a strong immune system. Once you have got a strong immune system carry on cleaning the rest of the organs such as the kidneys, lymph and skin. How do you detox the colon? There are many ways to clean all the organs. I think the simplest one is to start with activated charcoal for your colon, taken before bed away from any food intake. Charcoal is a strong chelator and can even detoxify the good nutrients you have just ate. Just mix a teaspoon with water and drink it for a couple of weeks at the same time eating clean food that does not create mucous. Mucous will just slow the whole system down and perhaps stop the cleanse altogether. A well-known liver cleanse is milk thistle. This herb supports the liver in doing its work and if you drink the lemon as well that helps the liver produce bile. The liver loves bitter so eating things like water-cress and kale will also help. Now you have the immune system sorted, move on to the kidneys. Uva Ersi, milk thistle, parsley juice with lemon, turmeric are all herbs that help the kidney. Eating less protein reduces the work load on the kidneys. The best way to clean the lymph is to jump on a trampoline because even the lymph from the ear lobes will be effected. Gravity squeezes the lymphatic vessels moving the lymph along. First thing when you get up jump on your trampoline for five minutes and then before bed jump on the trampoline for another 5 minutes. Movement moves your lymph because there is no lymph pump. How to cleanse your skin is as simple as eating water rich vegetables especially celery, drinking loads of water, cutting out the sugar, soya and coffee. Eat healthy fats like coconut, flax seeds, chia seeds, hemp seeds and avocados. Any toiletries or makeup has to be edible. If you can't eat it, don't put it on your skin.

**Minimize Stress**

We all know that stress is not beneficial to us. There are two types of stress; one is distress, which is damaging and u-stress is a good type of stress where you are really motivated to get things done and this type of stress can push you to do what you need without it being damaging.

We need to protect ourselves and our children from the distress. Adults naturally try to keep children from stressful situations because of adverse childhood reactions (ACE's) which can be anything from being bullied, parent illness, neglect, abuse, violence in the family, and many more have an impact across their whole life. The effect of unresolved emotional trauma from childhood on health across a lifetime is possibly the most underexposed risk factor for all major chronic health conditions in the world today. Huge studies by the CDC and Kaiser Permanente starting with 17,000 adults in the mid 1990's confirm stunning statistics.

Another part of minimizing stress is forgiving anyone who you feel a grievance towards because that person is probably not bothered about you, probably not even thinking about you, but if you are holding these feelings of revenge, you are the only one who will get ill. It is like drinking poison and expecting the other person to die and this is very damaging to your liver.

### What were you put on this Earth for?

Find your purpose in life because if you don't have a reason to live, life can be pointless. Even knowing what your life's purpose is gives you something to think about or work towards. When I say a purpose I mean how can you serve other people doing something that you are passionate about, so much so that it doesn't feel like work because you love it so much? Isn't that a fantastic position to be in? To never work a day in your life. Most people do not enjoy their job and because of the amount of time we spend working, about 1/3 of our life, this is a long time to be doing something that you don't enjoy.

Made in the USA
Columbia, SC
20 March 2018